Praise

"A fascinating look at the life of a strong resilient woman whose life was shattered by a car accident. Her spunk and petulance during rehabilitation will drive the reader to laughter despite the tragic circumstances... a must read for those who think they've been dealt a bad hand in life."
Dr. Fawzia Mail Tung

"Debra's sense of humor when talking about putting herself back together is refreshing. Readers will see how someone who had the rug pulled out from under her rose to new heights and didn't let her handicaps deter her from bettering the lives of others."
Nazli Currim, AUTHOR

"Debbie's story is one of resilience, persistence, healing and a commitment to community service. Her experience drives home how life can change in the blink of an eye and how it can either dig you into a hole or how you can climb your way up... reminds us that there is no better way to heal than by giving to others."
Sandy Bahr, Grand Canyon Director of the Sierra Club

"Hairy days in New York City as a social worker to a serious car accident in upstate NY that led to harrowing times in rehabilitation."
Barbara Fazio McGrory, CAC, SOCIAL WORKER

About the Author

A 1994 car accident ended Debra's career due to a traumatic brain injury. She re-invented herself through volunteer work and writing. Debra wrote for *Animal Wellness, Arizona Republic, Social Work, Airports of the World, Psychology Today,* and others. She reviewed books, contributed book chapters, and wrote a book for TFH Publications.

debrawhite.org

ALL SHOOK UP

Debra J. WHITE

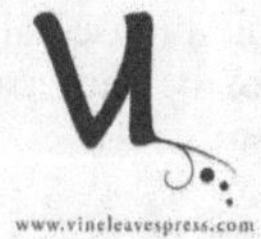

www.vineleavespress.com

Introduction

In 1982, I quit smoking and swore off junk food. No more cookies, hot dogs, cake, candy, donuts, ice cream, or washing down four White Castle burgers with a Coke. My stomach and my teeth thanked me. Four years earlier, I puffed my last joint and put alcohol behind me. That was the end of throbbing headaches the morning after. I swore that my head was used for batting practice. Instead of bar-hopping after work with a cigarette in one hand and a cocktail sloshing in the other, I took up jogging. At first, I could barely sweat through a mile having smoked for about twelve to thirteen years. Gasping for air with each step, my lungs took a beating but I persisted, forcing myself out of bed in the morning. On icy cold days, it was a challenge to leave the comfort of a warm bed but I did. Eventually, I logged many miles, mostly in New York City's Central Park. In 1985, I found a stray dog, who I named Scottie after my favorite Star Trek character, and he became my buddy and my running partner. If the weather permitted, Scottie trotted along at my side. In the 1990s, I biked up mountains in the Colorado Rockies, huffing and puffing as I pushed myself uphill hoping my water supply and energy bars would last. I backpacked in state parks in the Finger Lakes region of central New York. Over the years, I ran in road races on weekends, competing in three New York City marathons and one biathlon. I took out gym memberships. I became a vegetarian. My good health was on a roll, a far cry from the wasted days of drinking, smoking cigarettes and marijuana. Fast forward to January 6, 1994. I walked my two dogs after work. Instead of serving their evening meal, I ended up in a trauma center in a critical condition. A careless driver ran me over, leaving me bleeding and unconscious in a ditch with a traumatic brain injury, a gash on my cheek, and broken bones. I came home two months later to a vastly different world. I didn't have health insurance but that's another long story. Thankfully friends took care of my dogs in my long absence. I would've been heartbroken if they were surrendered to a shelter.

At the end of a long recovery, I had hard choices to make. I could sit home and become angry about what happened or I could find a new way to connect with the world around me. I'd always led an active life so I took on a variety of volunteer roles. Some were more interesting than others. Others challenged me in ways I didn't expect. A few made me feel tearful and sad. Many uplifted me. If the accident never happened, and sometimes I wish it didn't, these volunteer experiences would've passed me by. I have no regrets about the car accident on January 6, 1994. Here's how it happened and what I did next.

Since I can't remember half of my inpatient stay, I reconstructed part of this book from medical records (which I still have) and input from friends. I perused the files I kept from the accident. Not every employee's name is available and I don't remember them all. For consistency, I have used pseudonyms.

Chapter One
The Accident

On January 6, 1994, I lived in the Finger Lakes region of central New York. That particular winter morning, I probably woke up early and took my two dogs, Judy and Maxine, outside. Both dogs were rescues. I sipped lifesaving coffee while they took care of business. Then, I dressed warmly for the frigid winter weather, leashed Judy, my younger dog, for our regular morning jog. In 1982, I quit smoking. To stay off tobacco, I took up running. What a wonderful change.

Maxine had aged so her jogging days were over. In 1988, I had paid two dollars for her from a drug dealer in the crumbling Bronx neighborhood where I once worked. The dealer tried to sell me crack cocaine but I ended up with a scabby dog instead. Both dogs meant a lot to me.

After a brisk morning romp around the area, I showered, ate breakfast, maybe wheat toast or cold cereal topped with fruit, then drove to work. That was how I began each morning. I worked as a temp at the time. My dream job was still elusive.

In the spring of 1982, the Fortune 500 company I had worked for announced a reduction in force. Surely, I couldn't be on the chopping block. I had glowing performance reviews over the years and steadily moved up the corporate ladder. This girl was on the move, reading business magazines like Forbes and Fortune. I carried a briefcase to look important even if I wasn't. I never thought I'd work anywhere else. At the time I was let go, I was a few credits shy of a bachelor's degree in business administration. The company, by the way, had footed the bill for much of my degree through the tuition assistance program. I ran into roadblocks right away to locate another corporate job. During the 1980s, young people with MBAs from prestigious schools like Yale, Harvard, and Dartmouth were heavily recruited. Not me. My degree from a city college couldn't compete. An employment agency sent me out on a few interviews but nothing panned out. One counselor even asked me why I had applied for work through her agency. I needed a job, not her attitude. To avoid the poor house, I enrolled in a six-week word processing course. I found a secretarial job right away at a hospital. My fast fingers saved the day. I had fallen off the corporate ladder.

Around December, 1983, I rode a city bus to meet friends who jogged regularly in Central Park. For safety, I often joined runners several times a week for group runs. About to exit the bus, I noticed a bus advertisement asking for volunteers to work in a child abuse prevention program. Perhaps that would drag me out of my boredom. I ripped off one of the cards and mailed it. Then I said to myself, what the heck do you know about child abusers? I ended up working as a parent-aide to a woman who had abused her children. What an eye-opening experience where I learned about institutional racism, poverty, and abuse. After nearly two and a half years as a volunteer, I felt inspired to become a social worker. What else could I do? Working as a medical secretary nearly lulled me to sleep every day, even if the salary paid my bills. I eventually earned a masters in social work but I wasn't sure I had made the right choice. Serious social and economic issues confronted me like teen pregnancy, homelessness, poverty, gangs, and more. I thought I could save the world but my dreams were quickly shattered by a harsh reality. Maybe I should've given my decision to leave the field more time. I could sometimes be impatient.

I had dreams to become a writer as a child. In grade school, I had a following for the corny stories I wrote in a newsletter. I should've pursued writing as a career but life got in the way. So, I sent away for catalogs about journalism schools and fine arts programs. I had hoped to enroll in the next year. Surely, admissions counselor would be impressed with my background and talents and invite me into their program. What if I added more debt to my student loan portfolio? Except it didn't happen that way.

At the end of my tedious work days in upstate NY, I returned home, took the dogs out for a quick walk, made dinner, and got behind my computer. If I wasn't in the mood to write, I read a book, called a friend, or watched television. My lackluster life changed forever during that evening walk with Judy and Maxine. A man driving a van ran me over. The impact sent me sailing through the air until I landed in a snowbank seventy-five feet later, according to the driver's estimation on the police report. Was he speeding, intoxicated, or not paying attention? I'll never know the truth because he blamed the whole thing on me. He said my dogs ran loose on the road, a claim later proved false. Neighbors found my dogs, leashes still around their necks. It doesn't matter. Only the driver and the Almighty really know the truth about what had happened.

The first ambulance on the scene lacked special braces to protect my neck and spinal cord, which could have been damaged. Thankfully, my neck was not. A second ambulance arrived about half hour later. Oddly enough, the snow pile surrounding my head likely reduced the swelling in my brain, sparing me further damage. Ice typically reduces swelling. Snow did the same for me in this case.

According to medical records, I arrived at the county medical center, the only hospital in the entire county, at 6:40 p.m., almost one hour after being hit and "barely breathing." The paramedics said, "No other injuries other than around the head and face." Both the paramedics and the emergency room staff evidently failed to notice my grossly swollen left hand and wrist, sites of multiple fractures. Another ER form said my hands only had "minor abrasions." Three metacarpals, commonly known as knuckles, on my left hand and my left wrist were badly fractured. I bled from a two-centimeter laceration on my left cheek, which they failed to suture. I wonder why? Was it my lack of health insurance?

The driver's insurance company, Metropolitan Life, covered part of my hospital bills. My automobile insurance company came up with the rest. They hedged but had no choice. More on the insurance debacle later. A lot more.

Neighbors and friends cared for Judy and Maxine in my long absence. Maybe it was the Almighty or maybe it was luck because pets in situations like this often end up in shelters. I would have been devastated if I came home and found that my dogs were gone, surrendered to a shelter.

The county hospital sent me to Arnot Ogden, the trauma center in the city of Elmira, about forty-five miles away. I have no memory of the ride, how long it took, or the people inside the ambulance. The bills were already piling up yet I was in no position to even care about the battle to pay them. At the time of the accident, I was among the millions of gainfully employed but uninsured Americans. I had inquired about health insurance but it was prohibitively expensive. I can only imagine what today's rates are. I earned just above minimum wage but it was too much to qualify for state aid. Student loans, rent, car payments, food, and living expenses took precedence over health insurance. At the age of thirty-nine, I was young and in great shape so I didn't worry about the lack of health insurance. I never expected to land in the ICU either with no memory of the admission or the stay.

Chapter Two
The Trauma Center

The intensive care unit of Arnot Ogden Medical Center in Elmira admitted me in critical condition later that night. One ER note said I was "semi-conscious with very limited mobility." I had to be out of it because I didn't squeal when the Foley catheter was inserted into my bladder, a procedure I hear is uncomfortable. I don't like pain, cringe having my teeth cleaned, tried to donate blood once and fainted. In case of an emergency, call someone else but don't rely on me to help.

A series of X-rays and CT scans showed, "markedly comminuted fractures," on my left hand in stark contrast with the observations made at the county hospital (minor abrasions). They immobilized my left hand and wrist in a cast and sutured my left cheek to stem the bleeding. The scar is still visible and my left hand was never the same.

The attending physician reviewed CT films from Tompkins and noted, "There is an area in the right frontal lobe which is suspicious for a parenchymal contusion." Another form said of my brain, "Soft tissue swelling." An ER doctor said, "Amazingly she has not had more findings than we are able to identify in the emergency department."

Not much changed over the next ten days in the ICU. I slept most of the time. Rousing me was difficult. Not even the sound of a dog vomiting could wake me. When awake, I was in a stupor. The nursing staff moved me from the bed to a chair every few hours presumably to avoid bed sores. Every time a therapist tried to get me to stand I crumbled. My rubbery legs wouldn't cooperate.

Staff bathed me, brushed my teeth, and administered medications. Some days I ate the meals but I lost my appetite. Food fell from my mouth like I was gagging. Maybe it just didn't taste good. Other days I refused to eat. Besides the fact most hospital food didn't linger on the palate, brain trauma diminished my sense of taste, a problem I sometimes have.

Nearly all head trauma patients face fluctuating moods. I did. Some nursing notes described me as "calm" and "cooperative." Other notes said I was "combative" and "used foul language." That didn't surprise me. I'm from NYC where salty language sometimes peppered my speech.

Co-worker Abby visited me and said I mumbled, "I'm getting out of here. Just wait." Even in my altered state I was sure the hospital wasn't a place I wanted to be. Who likes to be in the hospital?

Of interest, friends brought my two dogs to visit me in the hospital. I have no recall whatsoever of their visits but medical records as well as my friends said that I correctly identified each dog. I slowly improved after their visits. The power of the human–animal bond is strong and powerful.

The car's impact smashed my brain against the tiny bony protrusions inside my skull. Brain cells and neurons were out of whack. The stupor controlled me. It would be another few weeks before my brain cooperated and my old self slowly reappeared.

Besides the brain contusion and fractured bones, CT scans showed a small lesion on my right ovary. No one at Arnot Ogden suggested I complete gynecological exam to evaluate the lesion. Car insurance only paid for injuries related to the accident and I had no health insurance. My ovaries weren't related to the accident. If the lesion was cancerous, I would've been stranded. Two years later when I qualified for Medicare, I went to a gynecologist and the lesion turned out to be benign. At least I escaped another medical catastrophe.

On January 17, I transferred to Highgate Manor, a rehab center about an hour away in Cortland, which treated patients with head trauma, mostly from accidents or strokes. That was ideal for me because I still had no idea where I was, what happened, or that I had a name.

Chapter Three
Highgate Manor

My mind turned into a torpedoed boat. The ship sputtered as it tried to stay afloat yet it refused to sink. A long time would pass before I realized how my brain was permanently altered. My own voyages would be limited and different from anything I had ever known.

A once thriving industrialized city, Cortland endured factory shut downs, home foreclosures, and small business failures. It was home to a unit of the state university. Outside the city, a network of meandering one-lane roadways crisscrossed undulating hills, towering pine trees, and green shrubs. The bucolic countryside didn't reflect the gritty times that pockmarked Main Street. I checked the current poverty rate in Cortland, which stands at about twenty-two percent. Seems like the city still faces challenges.

Highgate Manor, a major employer, was a squat, two-story, red brick building with a tired institutional look and the typical antiseptic smell of a healthcare facility. That would be my new home for a while.

I don't remember the ambulance drive or the admission process, even though my records indicated I knew my name. Though if someone called me Madonna, the tooth fairy, or Big Bird I may have also responded.

To evaluate incoming patients, Highgate utilized the services of Dr. John Cook (more on him later), one of two neurologists in Tompkins County. If the doctor was a quack or had the bedside manners of Godzilla, that was my tough luck. I had no say in who treated me.

Dr. Cook described me as "alert, oriented" while at the same time, the staff said I was only oriented to person. I remember nothing. My inner world still hemmed me in.

Notes written by occupational therapist Linda Sebastian on January 27 contradicted Dr. Cook's findings. Linda said, "Pt. does not appear to be oriented 3x. Attention span is poor. The pt. appears confused." I remember nothing of these evaluations.

Highgate filmed patients shortly after admission. Many patients were involved in accidents and films proved to be significant proof to stubborn insurance companies reluctant to pay claims for injured patients. Anyone who viewed my film would never describe me as "alert and oriented." I acted like someone sloshed on drugs or alcohol. I still have the video.

As my surroundings gradually became more familiar, I felt puzzled. Nothing looked familiar. I felt out of sorts, like waking up from a bad dream. I realized I wasn't home yet I wasn't sure where I was. In earlier days, too much alcohol gave me similar feelings. Thankfully, I quit drinking a long time ago. I had enough of ocean sized hangovers.

Without a memory to guide me, I had no idea what happened. The obvious canine telltale signs to remind me of home, such as a half-chewed rawhide bone or a slobbery squeak toy, were absent. So I searched for hints of my daily running habit. Again, I came up empty. No smelly running shoes or dirty socks. Something was wrong. It had to be Alzheimer's disease. My father had Alzheimer's that landed him in a nursing home before he died. He wasn't always coherent and neither was I. I didn't remember being hit by a car so that made sense.

Earlier that morning, an aide popped into my room and asked, "Do you remember what happened to you?"

The cast on my left hand dend wrist, the prominent scar on my left cheek, or the restraints holding me in bed failed to bring me to reality. "I have Alzheimer's disease, for crying out loud. Stop annoying me."

"You were hit by a car."

"I most certainly was not." Idiots worked at this place.

The aide mentioned my confusion to the staff psychologist, Dr. Nick Bella. After a few talks, I let go of the delusion only to get Dr. Bella off my back. I still had no concept of traumatic brain injury, a diagnosis that would follow me for the rest of my life.

I then noticed company in my room. I glanced at a middle-aged woman in the next bed. In typical New York City fashion, I asked, "Hey, yo, what's your name?"

"Rosie."

"What happened?"

Rosie stared blankly into space and spoke with slurred speech. "Got hit by a plane. Standing on the runway."

I envisioned a careless pilot running down a passenger waiting on the tarmac to board a small plane. I asked, "How long have you been here?"

Shrugging, Rosie said, "Years."

Crossing a dangerous intersection, Rosie's mid-sized car had been broadsided by a driver in a beefy pick-up who barreled through a stop sign. Rosie held death's doorknob and peered inside. Miraculously, the door slammed shut in front of her. By the time I got to Highgate, Rosie had been a patient for two and a half months. She spent six weeks in a coma attached to a respirator. Probably to her, the confinement felt like years.

Adjusting to institutional life at Highgate almost hammered me. At the age of thirty-nine, no one was about to tell me what to do, when to get up, and what to eat. I couldn't quite grasp why I needed help. The world around me shattered and I couldn't cobble the broken pieces back together. As a social worker, I helped people. I never expected to be in a position where I needed help myself. I wasn't thrilled either.

Our day started somewhere between 6:30 and 7:00 a.m., depending on which side of the floor the aides got to first. If there was only one woman on duty, the wait for a sponge bath could be a while. At home, I showered every morning but the effect of hospitalization hadn't caught up with me yet. I probably had pasty skin from being inside so long, but I wasn't at a point to care.

When our turn came, two female aides burst into our room and flipped on the overhead lights. The sharp glare from fluorescent bulbs made my eyes squint. Brain trauma also caused light sensitivity. I craved dark sunglasses or an umbrella to shield the glare. In addition, because of the almost intoxicating effects of Phenobarbital to prevent epileptic seizures—it didn't work—I woke up every day feeling loopy, almost like having a hangover.

Once I sat up and hid from the glare, an aide filled a wash basin with tepid water and placed it on the table next to my bed. As soon as she zipped the curtain around me, she handed me a wash cloth and a bar of soap. I felt ashamed that a strange woman had to assist me. I could barely undress. I glanced down at my bare breasts and used my good arm to cover them up.

"Stop looking," I said.

"Everyone, including you, has to be supervised during a bath. Rules are rules."

"At least turn around."

"No, I can't."

"Then I won't wash," I said.

The disgruntled aide finally caved in and I finished my sponge bath. We went through this routine for a few days until I finally accepted it was now part of my day.

Rosie, on the other hand, seemed to take it all in her stride, but not me. For most of my life, I was fiercely independent. I jogged at dawn and worked a full-time job. At times, I worked two jobs because of the punishing costs of rent, utilities, food, credit cards, and student loans. I earned both my undergraduate and graduate degrees part-time. Even when I became seriously ill with chicken pox at the age of thirty-three, I took care of myself. I had been a volunteer at a homeless family shelter. An outbreak of chicken pox didn't concern me. I assumed I had the virus as a child. Turns out I did not and I got very sick.

Suddenly, I was a member of a very distinct club, one I would've preferred not to join. I was tied to my wheelchair, tied to my bed at night, and at the mercy of others. I was in a full-blown snit. Get me out of here.

Making me feel worse, the aides picked out my clothing, usually sweatpants and a long-sleeved T-shirt. Normally, I was a fastidious dresser. Even my socks had to match my outfits. Most of my wardrobe came from second hand stores in ritzy neighborhoods. My nose sniffed out sharp looking outfits at cheap prices. Now, I wasn't concerned about what I wore. Those of us who walked with assistance wore high-top sneakers, supposedly to help prevent ankle injuries if we stumbled.

After I freshened up, an aide guided me into my wheelchair. She whisked me to the bathroom, lifted me onto the bowl and stared at me, with her arms folded. When I was dazed, the lack of privacy wasn't an issue. I was aghast the aide now expected me to take a dump with her standing in front of me. A few things in life demand privacy and bowel elimination is one of them. I developed constipation because I refused to crap in front of strangers. I waited until later in the day when friends visited. One of them stood outside until I was done.

Once the morning routine was over, an aide secured my wheelchair straps because I was so wobbly. If not assisted, I tumbled to the floor. Injured brain tissue doesn't rejuvenate by itself so easily. Other parts of the brain kick in and take over the work of damaged areas. The brain doesn't work as well as it used to. Although I had no serious leg injuries, the signals from my brain to my legs weakened, compromising my ability to walk. Patients like Rosie with severe head trauma needed more time and assistance to learn how to walk again. Some never regained that function.

The dual-purpose wheelchair restraints stopped me from hurting myself. After admission, a newly hired aide inadvertently left me unrestrained. Without thinking, I got up and promptly landed on the floor. Maybe in my warped mind I saw this as a chance to escape and go home. Nothing serious happened to me other than a few bumps and bruises. From that point on, I was restrained unless a staff member was present. The restraints also protected Highgate from negligence suits.

Restraints, however, made me feel trapped like in a strait jacket. The second the aide walked out, I wiggled, squirmed, and twisted, trying to free myself. Confinement was hard to handle. Throughout the day, I seized every available chance to unfasten the straps. Highgate must've been prepared because no matter how hard I picked and pulled, I never broke free.

Orderlies carrying breakfast trays showed up sometime each morning after we were dressed. Food lost its appeal. In addition to my dull taste buds, the eggs were most often cold and runny, the toast was soggy, and the muffins of unknown origin were usually drier than scouring powder. I temporarily forgot I started the day with a cup of coffee and reading the *Times*. I bypassed breakfast and waited for the first round of rehabilitation to begin.

Rosie and I started talking during quiet moments. I couldn't make out everything she said, but I listened. Rosie had acquired a severe speech impediment. She was having a hard time, just like me. Even though our communication was tricky, Rosie and I connected. We shared a strong bond and stayed friends for a while. Over the years, we lost touch. I always hoped that she had a good life.

During the lull, I often gazed out the window at mounds of snow piled in the parking lot. I felt out of sorts, unfamiliar with my new world. Delusions taunted me. I thought I lived in a house with two floors. It only had one. I swore Highgate rested on a sprawling green golf course. The building was surrounded by iron gray cement. I heard voices that I didn't trust. I drifted in between my brain wobbled world and reality. It seemed easier to cope when my imagination convinced me I was the CEO of a major Fortune 500 company and not a patient in a rehab center. I was scared, frustrated, and unsure what would become of me.

Chapter Four
Therapy, Therapy, and More Therapy

Brain trauma impacted my memory. I retained a solid block of long-term memory with some gaps here and there. My short-term memory, however, took a wallop. I felt robbed, cheated, and stung by simple things I couldn't remember any more. Even if they were unimportant, I wanted to make that decision, but I couldn't. Thoughts, simple ideas, and memories drifted away. No matter how hard I chased them, they turned into grains of sand slipping through my grasp.

A whirlwind of employees buzzed around the facility all day—occupational therapists, cognitive therapists (I didn't know what they did), psychologists, social workers, orderlies, nurse's aides, nurses, and doctors. I could barely remember my own name. Now I was supposed to remember another long list of strange people and the role each played in my recovery. Probably everyone explained their purpose but no one made much sense. I wasn't even sure I liked all these people. Housekeeping and food service staff also breezed in and out mopping floors or delivering meals. All the foot traffic and noise overwhelmed me. I tried to cope with congregate care. My strings were still loose, however.

From my bed, I glanced outside at the steely gray clouds one morning, waiting for therapy to begin. An aide stepped in and asked, "Do you know where you are?"

Why ask me such a ridiculous question. "I'm at Arnot Ogden Medical Center in Elmira," I said, snapping to attention.

The aide's scrunched up face said I was wrong. "You're in Highgate Manor in Cortland."

That was it. For all I knew, Highgate could've been a meat packing plant or a pickle factory. "No, I'm not."

The back and forth continued until I accepted the change of venue. Nothing about Arnot Ogden was familiar, but something must've seeped into my brain because I insisted I was still there. I'm a New Yorker and most native New Yorker's are paranoid and suspicious about something or another. Every stranger could be a potential thief, scam artist, or axe murderer. I viewed the staff at Highgate with the same suspicion. Something wasn't right and I didn't like it. I wasn't sure how the staff expected me to cooperate when I couldn't trust them. To me, they were all strangers.

Of course, I didn't need rehabilitation. How dare someone attach a daily schedule to my wheelchair so I would know where and when to go for each group? That was the ultimate insult to a woman with a master's degree from a respected private university and who read the *New York Times*. The *Times* for crying out loud. Now, someone else had my days planned. I could only take so much.

"What's this?" I asked, trying to rip off the plastic cover and shred it to pieces.

"Your schedule," the aide said.

I was absolutely indignant. "Don't need a schedule."

"Yes, you do. Everyone does."

"I'd rather stay in my room," I said. "Not in the mood for rehab."

"Patients attend groups, except the people on ventilators."

The swift changes baffled me. There was a cast on my left arm so the aides placed my watch on my right wrist. Cripes, I couldn't get used to that. Time had no meaning anyway. I mean, like, where was I going? To Austria for an Alpine ski vacation? The impact shattered my glasses so I wore a pair with an old prescription. Naturally, I had trouble seeing. I'd worn glasses since the third grade.

Rehab was my only ticket to freedom so, begrudgingly, I cooperated. Not because my injuries were serious but only to get out of Highgate.

But nothing came easy. Confused and bewildered, I either pushed myself to another patient's room or rode the elevator to the wrong floor. I couldn't get the hang of the routine at Highgate. I just wanted to go home.

The current events therapist grumbled at my frequent blunders.

"Don't you know how important groups are?"

Connie made it seem as if the current events group, of which I had just missed half, was a life or death situation. To me, however, what was happening in the outside world, namely the massive earthquake that rocked southern California and the winter Olympics in Lillehammer, Norway, was of little concern. I felt humiliated by her admonishment but refused to let her know.

"What's the big deal?" I said with a shrug.

"Don't miss my group," Connie said.

"I got lost on the way."

"Try harder next time."

"Yeah, yeah, yeah."

•

Physical therapy was even more of a challenge, even though I was lean and athletic from years of running and biking. I thought it would be a breeze. Nope. It was not. Being in shape and eating a healthy diet probably sped up my recovery, but nothing came easily.

Patients met in a huge, well-lit room with exercise machines, treadmills, leg weights and stationary bikes, but this was no ordinary gymnasium. No broad chested men pumping iron or middle-aged women working off a little cellulite were around. The rehab scene reminded me of a fairy tale. We were all a Humpty Dumpty piecing ourselves back together again.

Sofia Munoz, my physical therapist, said, "Today, we work on safety."

I thought she referred to self-defense methods in case a mugger attacked me. Brain damaged people sometimes interpret statements literally. Ted Bundy, the serial murderer, might be taken for a man who hacked apart boxes of breakfast cereal.

"I'm safe, aren't I?" I wondered if we had to protect ourselves against dangerous interlopers who lurked in the shadows.

"That's not quite what I mean," Sofia said. "We'll go over transferring from the wheelchair to the exercise table."

That may seem like an ordinary routine, but to me it was more exasperating than the day I competed in a biathlon and transferred from a bike to running shoes in mere seconds then took off for the running part of the competition. I finished, by the way.

For safety, Sofia constantly needled me to secure the wheelchair brakes before standing. After a while, I got sick of the reminders. She opened each session with the same question, "What's first?"

I usually forgot the brakes existed. Up until the accident, I was never in a wheelchair. Mastering proper wheelchair use exhausted me.

If I didn't respond correctly with, "Put the brakes on," Sofia waggled her finger at me and repeated the correct response. In the end, the message sunk in.

I progressed to table exercises such as rollovers and sit ups. Because of the cast on my left arm, push-ups, or other exercises to build upper body strength were impossible. The goal was to advance me to a walker or a cane. For someone who had run in at least seventy-five road races, including three marathons, I now felt wiped out and washed up. What would become of me?

Since I refused to eliminate in front of the aide, the urge sometimes caught up to me during morning physical therapy. Each therapist supervised two to three patients at the same time.

Hoping to catch Sofia off guard, I said, "I have to go to the bathroom." Busy supervising a newly admitted patient I figured she'd let me sit on the bowl for a few minutes by myself. No such luck. Disappointed, Sofia rested her arm behind the bathroom sink and waited for me to go. I wouldn't.

I graduated to stair climbing. As Sofia gripped the side of my slacks, I trudged up a short flight of stairs, using my cane for balance. Going up took forever and coming down almost didn't happen. I wanted to cheat and ride the elevator. The downward motion always felt as if I would tumble and roll down the stairs. Thankfully, I never did.

Every step was painstakingly slow. My legs, especially the left one, felt like slabs of stone. They never felt that bad when I ran long distances, including the punishing 26.2 miles of the New York City marathon. Walking a straight line was nearly impossible. I would've easily flunked a field sobriety test. Naturally, I wanted to sit down to rest. I wondered if I would always feel like this. And I still had no understanding as to why a crushing blow to the head hampered my ability to walk. None of the staff explained it to me either. Or if they did, I don't remember.

•

Besides a physical therapy group every day, there was occupational therapy. Originally, I thought occupational therapy (OT) was related to employment training. Indeed, I wanted a more demanding job than the one I no longer had but I didn't think now was the time to deal with it. In fact, employment seemed elusive for most of us. OT had nothing to do with employment training but introduced disabled people to independent living skills. I couldn't believe that someone had to show me how to use cutlery again.

Unlike the old days when disabled people, especially children, depended on family or caregivers, the current philosophy advocated maximum freedom and independence. Disabled people were taught activities of daily living with minimal or no outside assistance. That sounded good to me. No way would strangers meddle in my life. I lived independently since 1976 and planned to keep it that way.

I didn't know how but I would brew my own coffee, bake my own bran muffins, and shop for sales as I always did. I had to get home for my dogs and scramble their eggs. Determined to crawl out of this calamity, no one would send me to a group home, which happened to some patients.

Linda Sebastian, the same therapist who disagreed with the neurologist when I was admitted, became my occupational therapist. The doctor said I was alert and oriented. Linda said I was confused and out of it. If I was the featured guest on the Oprah Show or danced with wolves on my admission to the center, I had no memory of it. I still don't.

During a session about eating habits, I was affronted when Linda said, "You eat too fast."

"Don't pick on me."

"You come across as sloppy. Slow down."

"I'm not a slob."

"I didn't say that, just take your time when you eat."

In another session, I used a spoon when I should've reached for a fork. I didn't see it as a big deal.

"Don't be in such a rush," she said.

"Leave me alone."

OK, I was touchy. I didn't appreciate a younger woman showing me how to eat. That I forgot how was a blow I couldn't handle. The therapist was doing her job. I shouldn't have given her a hard time.

Another day, Linda scrunched up her nose and said, "Your hand and arm smell."

I felt insulted. "Can't help it," I said, nodding at my cast.

Obviously, I couldn't wash from the elbow down so my skin probably reeked.

"Follow me," Linda said.

With a dampened wash cloth, she wiped down each of my fingers. Linda seemed delighted with her little chore and broke into a wide grin. "Isn't that better?"

Appreciative I wasn't even though the rank odor was gone. Confinement was killing me and undoubtedly it showed. It was time to swallow my pig-headed pride if I wanted to go home.

•

Once a licensed social worker myself, cognitive therapy was new to me. The entire concept sounded hokey. Cognitive therapy retrained brain injured patients in such areas as memory, concentration, and proper vocabulary usage.

By the end of January, I read at the third grade level. My brain was like a wilted bowl of fruit, even though I once read classics by Shakespeare, Dickens, and Tolstoy. I devoured books of all kinds and amassed a huge collection at the time of the accident. Now I had little recollection of these important works. My interest in reading had all but vanished. I was afraid I'd be like this forever. People would think I had the intellect of a mole.

The cognitive therapist, Emily Blakewell, was a former grade school teacher. She was a pleasant young woman with an easy smile and cool blue eyes. I liked her right away. Maybe this fueled my motivation to pick up the pace.

My mind was a spongy mess because I couldn't remember word lists Emily read to me. Simple math confounded me too. Accounting stumped me in college. I almost failed but passed with a D. Phew, what a relief. At one time I managed a medium-sized credit union. Emily assured me I would improve, but I was doubtful. If I couldn't read beyond a third grade level and perform grammar school arithmetic, I would never get beyond Highgate. No wonder Emily's notes said I was frustrated. The idea of being institutionalized scared the hell out of me. That would mean a life with no dogs, no morning coffee, or dragging a week's worth of dirty clothes to the corner laundry. I'd have to live with someone watching over my shoulder all the time. That couldn't happen.

One day, Emily handed me a sheet of paper resembling a checkbook. My bill paying task ended in a bust. I couldn't figure out how much to pay my creditors. Subtracting ten from fourteen was beyond me. My irritation level surged past the boiling point when I shredded the paper and hurled the pieces on the floor. I pushed myself out, knocking my chair into the door as I left in haste. Later, Emily stopped by my room and said, "We'll try again tomorrow. It's hard on some patients." That small gesture stretched a long way.

The next morning, Emily placed a straightforward map in front of me with instructions to start at point A and end at point B. That, too, frazzled me. Handling directions frazzled me to the point of tears.

They still do. GPS helps but I still get lost. That session ended, though, without me having an outburst. Emily urged patience. That would be hard because nothing in my background prepared me for this. Who in New York City had patience?

In addition to physical, occupational, and cognitive therapy, I had mental health therapy with a twenty-something social worker named Nancy O'Leary. Two psychologists worked at Highgate and I had already developed a rapport with Dr. Bella, the man who tried to convince me Alzheimer's disease wasn't my problem. I didn't want mental health therapy at all yet if I had to, I preferred Dr. Bella. I don't remember how this was resolved because I ended up having sessions with Nancy twice a week.

One of the first questions that Nancy asked was, "How do you feel?"

I should've remembered this introduction from social work school. Instructors drilled students to ask this question to clients when discussing emotions. Once I graduated in 1988, I landed a job in the South Bronx, a poor neighborhood rife with gangs, violence, and abandoned buildings. I felt like small when I asked my first client, "how do you feel?" The single mother of four scraped by on a measly welfare check and resided in a rat-infested tenement asked me for a food voucher. Of course, she was desperate and about to go crazy living in abject poverty. If I lived under those conditions, I would've jumped off the Brooklyn Bridge.

Thoughts raced through my mind in therapy that morning. How the heck would Nancy feel if she just lost her independence? If she was in diapers at the age of thirty-nine? Diapers that I couldn't change. If she had strangers next to her while she sat on the toilet? I wasn't in the mood to talk to someone else about my life. Enough was enough. I spent all day interacting with people I didn't know, some of whom pestered me. I wasn't used to talking about myself so much. I wanted out.

"Get me out of here," I said. "I'll like you better."

"We're here to talk about you. Talking may help you feel better."

I was sick of talking and slammed my good hand against the table. "How?"

Nancy casually checked her watch. Then, she looked at me with a raised eyebrow. "We have forty-three minutes left. Start by telling me what's on your mind."

Oblivious to my simmering anger, she explained I wasn't ready for discharge yet. Oh yes, I was. What'd she know. I became further agitated when she said I had to undergo more rehabilitation before discharge. As far as I was concerned, I had all the rehab I needed.

A few sessions passed and I stopped seething. I confided in Nancy just a bit. "I can't remember the names of friends who visit me. I'm embarrassed to ask who they are. And now I'm pissed off at the driver. Why didn't he see my two dogs and me? I want to slide my feet into a pair of running shoes and go for a brisk jog. I don't care how cold it is outside."

Jogging kept me grounded in the wacky world of New York City. Bad luck always happened to other people, not me. During my thirty-five-year tenure in the Big Apple, I never confronted a crime more serious than a stolen bicycle or a pervert groping my behind on a crowded subway. I wasn't sure how I could handle the aftermath of the accident.

Shortly after I began therapy, Nancy offered a suggestion. "How about group therapy? It might help."

Just when I didn't think I could take another shred of therapy, I sat inside a support group meeting for head injured patients. Before the first session began, I was sure I'd hate it. To shut my therapist up, I agreed to attend one meeting.

For the first time, I shared space with brain injured patients who had broken lives and broken bodies like me. A few were elderly who pulled through debilitating strokes. One man toppled off a three-story building at a construction site. Drunk drivers plowed into a few patients leaving them with grave injuries. Now people are brain injured from drivers texting behind the wheel. Brain damage had wide-reaching effects on the body and mind.

The head injury group met daily and I attended most meetings. Talking with other patients was more therapeutic than individual therapy. Brain damage was permanent—something the rehab therapists never told me. If they did, I forgot. Spending time with the group threw me off the pity pot. At least I could talk, which was more than a lot of them could do. I may have missed words and confused sentence structure but at least I could blab my big mouth. That was a small comfort for a shameless agitator like me.

One young woman, with severe frontal lobe damage, barely contained her emotions. She ranted and raved, hurling vile epithets at everyone. "Fuck you," the woman said to the therapist.

"Please, no foul language," O'Leary, the group leader, said.

"I'll curse if I want to. You can't stop me."

In all the years I lived in New York City, I sometimes cursed and swore at people who irritated me, including drug dealers who hawked crack in front of my apartment building or the men who made lewd passes at me as I left Central Park in running shorts on hot humid afternoons.

I felt sorry for the woman with temporal lobe damage because she became the group pariah. No one, including me, wanted anything to do with her. She lashed out at everyone.

Another young man with an active life now dealt with tremors. His speech was slurred. He probably would require round-the-clock care. That could've been me but it wasn't.

An elderly stroke patient named Helen spoke about her fears. "Can I make it when I leave? I'm scared I'll need care for the rest of my life."

"You seem strong enough that you can manage," someone said.

"Don't let them send me to the nursing home," Helen said, voice cracking. "I want to go home."

Soon, she launched into sobs. I was sorry for the gray-haired woman as tears streamed down her cheeks.

"Helen, if people don't like the way you look, the heck with them," I said. "Do the best you can. Be strong."

Helen dabbed her puffy eyes with a tissue. She cracked a faint smile. "I don't like people talking bad about me because I talk funny now."

"Tell them to back off, you're a goddess."

Helen cracked up. So did everyone else. We had a good laugh that day and Helen left with a smile on her face.

I made someone laugh again, like I used to. That was a sign I made progress. Someday soon, I would leave Highgate and resume my life. Helen felt better that day and so did I.

Chapter Five

Life in Rehab

I remained convinced my new roommate Rosie had been hit by a plane. She was still out of it, forgetting that she attended college. Crazy thoughts and words drifted between us. Not everything made sense yet our bond slowly built. At night before lights out, we talked but who knows about what?

One morning Rosie and I chatted after breakfast. "You like the head injury group?" I asked.

Rosie threw her head back and boasted, "Don't have a head injury."

"Oh my, I'm sorry. What'd you have then?"

"Dunno."

I had no idea what was wrong with her either. That should've served as a sign I still had cat litter scrambling around my brain. Of course, Rosie had a head injury, a very serious one. The collision with the pick-up nearly killed her. Every patient at Highgate Manor had some type of brain trauma whether from a stroke, accident, or illness.

·

With each day, I became more with it. I soon developed a beef with the graveyard shift. Highgate scheduled only a handful of employees for the overnight hours. Why, I wasn't sure. Maybe to save money. Highgate after all was a for profit facility. Employees blabbed through the empty halls to stay in touch. The shouting often roused me from sleep yet Rosie was unmoved. She slept through everything. I expected yelling for emergencies but I resented yapping about soap operas and boyfriends at 2:00 a.m. Phenobarbital and a full day of therapy wiped me out. I needed my beauty rest to recover. Complaining to a supervisor about the midnight clatter was pointless. Hardly anyone listened to us patients anyway.

Take Rosie's ear-ache for example. She complained repeatedly to staff about an itchy, painful ear. She scratched her ear and shook her head all the time. Everyone ignored her until the infection was so severe that surgical ear drainage was needed.

•

Incontinence added to my new set of woes. Once the Foley catheter was removed, I wore adult diapers. Imagine me, at age thirty-nine, in diapers. Although outgoing, I was modest in other ways. I rarely undressed in front of strangers. If I had suddenly regained my senses, I would've been mortified knowing that staff saw me naked, some of whom I didn't even like.

As a way to wean me off diapers, two aides who I called the potty patrol, escorted me to the bathroom every two hours. I wasn't thrilled to be woken up in the middle of the night, dumped into my wheelchair, and plopped on the toilet while two strange women stared at me.

"Leave me alone," I said, wiping sleep from my eyes.

"Use the bathroom."

"Don't have to."

The aides were persistent. "Doctor's orders say you're supposed to go."

"What if I can't?"

"Squeeze it out."

One night, I slipped and wet the bed. That annoyed the potty patrol because they had to change my linens and clean my wet pajamas. Humiliated that I urinated on myself, tears ran down my cheeks as the staff changed the sheets and handed me a dry gown to wear. I hadn't lost control of my bladder since my wild and wacky partying years that ended in 1978.

The head nurse paid me a visit the next morning. "Use the call button on your bed," she said, "or it's back to diapers."

She pointed to the small, cream-colored buzzer.

"I forget sometimes."

"Try to remember."

Nights with the potty patrol helped me to master bathroom training. Free of adult diapers forever, there would be no more strangers demanding that I urinate on demand at the midnight hour. Or so I hoped.

•

Brain trauma initially affected my social skills. Except for my relationship with Rosie, I hardly socialized with other patients, highly unusual for me. In second grade, I received a D in conduct because I ran my mouth so often. As president of my high school I addressed audiences all the time. I chatted with dog owners in my West Side neighborhood. Reserved and quiet would not describe me. Now I didn't want to talk to anyone, especially to strangers. They made me uncomfortable.

Dr. Bella, the psychologist, caught me leaving a therapy group. To bolster my people skills, he said, "You'll eat lunch today in the cafeteria."

The heck I would.

The injury also dampened my taste. My mouth felt dry all the time. Add that to utter exhaustion from anti-seizure drugs and I stopped eating the midday meal. At noon almost every day, I returned to my room, asked an aide to help me in bed and I slept for the hour. How dare he suggest I eat with strangers? "I'd rather sleep than eat."

Dr. Bella stood his ground. "Time you socialized with the others."

"No."

Next thing you know, I sat at an empty table with four place settings. The tidy dining room had a pleasant feel but nothing that would make the centerfold for *Better Homes and Gardens*. Regardless, I didn't want to be there. As Dr. Bella was ready to leave, he tapped my shoulder and said, "I'll stop by your room later to see how things went."

"I'm not staying."

"Have fun." He grinned on his way out.

By the time Dr. Bella was out of sight, two other patients took their places at the table. One made casual conversation but I acted aloof. The very second a staff member served our meals I zipped my wheelchair around and pushed myself back to my room. No one was telling me what to do.

Although Rosie ate in the dining room almost daily, I was unmoved. I could've easily joined her but I balked. Frightened about ending up in a group home, I couldn't bear the idea of living among strangers. I spurned eating with them, too. That was my one and only foray into the dining room. I wanted to be home, eating my own food, playing with my dogs, and doing whatever I wanted.

I missed dressing for work, rifling through my closet and swearing I had nothing to wear. During the years I rode the NYC subway, I always read a newspaper, book, or magazine. My social life included after work dinners, movies, plays, and museum exhibits. Rehab was now my full day of work.

My defiance extended to another group (therapeutic rehabilitation) that I flatly rejected. The group leader was supposed to help patients regain interest in their hobbies. No college kid would show me how to regain interest in long distance jogging and reading the *New York Times*. A terse note in my medical record said, "Pt. refuses TR group." I never figured out why I blew off TR.

·

Twice a week, all patients showered. Good thing I was in a slump because I bathed daily, even when my Manhattan studio churned out ice-cold water. Without a daily shower, I felt grungy. An aide helped me out of bed and to take off my clothes. That humiliated me because I could hardly accept the impersonal nature of institutional life. Once naked, I sat in my wheelchair while the aide covered me with a large piece of flimsy cotton material, about the size of a bed sheet.

"What kind of chintzy rag is this?"

"To keep you covered until we get to the shower."

"Everyone will know I'm naked underneath," I said, certain staff and patients could see my behind.

"Hurry, my butt is cold."

The aide giggled. "Here we go."

I should've lightened up but I didn't.

Behind closed doors, the aide threw off the privacy cloth. She turned on the shower, handed me a bar of soap, and whisked me underneath warm water cascading out of the spout. Because of the cast on my left arm, I needed help washing. I felt so exposed having a stranger shampoo my hair. The flowing water covered up my unhappy tears. By the time the shower was over, my spasms of sorrow were no longer visible.

Talking about my fears and concerns in therapy groups may have helped but I never gave it a chance. If the staff saw me as weak they'd never let me leave. So I threw up a barrier that said nothing bothered me. I was going home, even though I had no career, no money, and no family close by and an uncertain future. There was a place for me somewhere in the world. I just wasn't sure how to find it. My dogs, however, depended on my recovery.

•

Early one morning, Rosie was out of sorts. When an aide waltzed in, Rosie pleaded for help. "I lost my mop."

Her quivering voice suggested desperation, but I wasn't sure why. I doubted cleaning our room was part of the rehabilitation program. The profit pounding healthcare companies wouldn't stoop that low, although it wouldn't surprise me if they did. After all, they boosted their bottom line by depriving vital healthcare from sick and injured people like us.

The aide gently squeezed Rosie's hand and asked, "What're you looking for?"

"My mop," red-faced Rosie pleaded. "Help me find it. Please."

Confused, I tried to remember if Rosie ever had a mop. If she had one, what color was it? Was it small or large? If I needed a mop, where was mine?

The puzzled aide peeked inside Rosie's small closet, allowing Rosie to watch. Perhaps the aide thought some article of clothing or other personal item would grab Rosie's attention. I hoped she wasn't honestly scrounging around for a mop.

Every time the aide said, "I don't see a mop," Rosie fussed.

Haggling went on for a few minutes yet Rosie remained distressed. When the aide suddenly left, I wheeled myself next to Rosie. "Did you really lose a mop?"

"I'm cold."

The aide returned with her supervisor. I nodded in Rosie's direction and said, "She's cold. I bet she wants a sweater." Once the nurse fished a thick wool sweater out of the closet and helped slide Rosie into it, the crisis ended. That I was able to end Rosie's predicament was a sign of my slow, steady improvement. My brain was slowly mending.

•

Most aides were decent people working for meager wages. Ever since the factories shifted overseas or to the non-union South, the supply of good paying jobs dried up too. I don't know how happy I'd be cleaning up someone's bowel movements, but to struggling people, Highgate was a paycheck. A few workers managed to smile and asked about our recovery. My thinking was disrupted and I probably never asked the workers how they were. Maybe they understood we weren't thoughtless or uncaring.

As my taste buds slowly re-awakened, I resumed my vegetarian diet, but meal requests not always honored. I shunned the mystery meat and picked at the limp, salty canned vegetables instead. If I was lucky, one of my friends brought me Chinese takeout or pasta salad. Otherwise, I skipped the tasteless institutional dinners. None of the aides objected to my picky eating, but all that changed one evening.

A burly young man with a neck the size of a tree trunk barreled into my room holding a dinner tray.

"Excuse me, I don't want anything."

Buzz cut snarled and said, "You're going to eat."

Those were fighting words. If I didn't want to eat, this miscreant certainly wasn't going to make me. "I don't want anything."

Veins bulged in his neck. "Eat this."

"No," I said. "You can't make me."

Then I got scared, wondering if he would rough me up because I was alone. Rosie was in the dining room. As I was about to wail, one of my friends walked in. When I noticed takeout Chinese food in her hand, I pointed to it and said, "She has my dinner." I wanted to hurl the tray at him and watch the food crawl down his back.

The hulk stormed out and I told my friend about his crude behavior. She marched to the nurse's station and that was the last time I ever saw him. I don't know if he was asked to leave or told to stay away from me. Either way, I didn't care. A heavy hand wasn't what I expected from a rehab worker.

•

A newly hired aide rolled me out of bed at 6:00 a.m. one morning for an off-site 10:00 a.m. medical appointment with an orthopedic doctor about my arm. I wondered why the early rise.

"Time to get up. You have a doctor's appointment," she said, smacking on a wad of pink bubble gum.

"Where, in Brooklyn Heights?"

After the standard wash up routine the aide strapped in my wheelchair. When the same aide served my breakfast, which I refused, I said, "Help me back to bed, please." Even though my anti-seizure dose was lowered, I was drowsy most of the time, especially in the morning.

Leaving an exhausted patient tied up in a wheelchair next to an empty bed was mean. It also pissed me off.

"You got to see the doctor."

"Look at the time? I'm cold. I want to get under the covers." An Arctic blast blanketed the area with sub-zero temperatures. Savage winds rocked the windows.

"Nope, you can't."

"I don't have anything else to do." I was excused from therapy groups that morning.

The unyielding aide sorted through my dirty clothes because it was laundry day. "I said you can't go back to bed."

That was the last straw. I screamed as if someone yanked my toenails off with pliers. When the aide approached my bed, I threw a pillow at her. Seconds later a nurse arrived and asked me what was wrong.

"I have a doctor's appointment at 10:00 a.m." I pointed at the aide and said, "She won't let me lay down. I'm tired and cold."

The nurse glanced at my untouched plate of food. "What about your breakfast?"

"She made me so upset I can't eat." OK, so I stretched it a bit.

The aide jumped in and said, "You said you were hungry."

"I never said that."

The nurse stood next to me. "Calm down." She glanced at the aide and said, "Go to the next room. I'll finish in here."

On her way out, the aide handed me a dirty look and I stuck out my tongue. The nurse agreed it was pointless for me to sit in the wheelchair for another three hours. She helped me into bed and I curled up under the covers, confused I had to act like a whack job in order to gain understanding.

In the past, I used humor to attract attention. This was the first time I resorted to hysteria. At least it worked.

•

Later that morning, the orthopedic doctor allowed his assistant to change my cast. The new one strangled my arm but my muddled mind didn't notice right away. Brain trauma still hid me under a cloud. When the doctor checked me over, he didn't see anything unusual either. A few hours later, the tips of my fingers swelled to the size of link sausages. I had trouble moving them. I complained to the staff, but everyone ignored me.

For the next two days, I endured puffy, painful fingers until I wheeled myself next to a sink full of water. I put my arm inside to rinse off the cast and that got attention. A nurse called the orthopedic doctor and he said to remove the cast. They replaced it with a removable splint. My fat fingers returned to normal size a few days later. The soreness from the impact persisted but at least my hand didn't feel like it had been steamrolled by a semi.

•

In mid-February, I inexplicably developed a red, scaly rash that started on my lower legs and slowly spread upwards to include my torso. To alleviate the itch, Dr. Freeman, the physician in charge, prescribed an anti-inflammatory cream, which the aides applied every few hours.

The next day, the rash spread covering most of my body. Ugly red, scaly patches were everywhere. No one consulted a dermatologist. Instead, Dr. Freeman prescribed Benadryl, an over-the-counter allergy medication, but the red, scaly patches worsened. The itch intensified. Then, a fever of unknown origin spiked to 103–104. I felt so debilitated. Rehab came to an abrupt standstill.

On an afternoon when my skin was on fire, Sofia, the physical therapist, appeared in my room. "Why aren't you in therapy?"

"Look at me, I'm sick."

"You shouldn't miss so much therapy. We have work to do," Sofia said.

I was so drained I could barely move.

"You're only hurting yourself by not coming," Sofia said as she spun around and left.

Like rehab would cure my itch and fever?

Dr. Freeman discussed my case with a small group of staff physicians. One suggested I was allergic to the anti-seizure medication. Another blamed the laundry detergent used on the sheets. The head nurse said she had no idea what was going on. Several possibilities existed. The rash and the fever were related. More likely, however, there were two distinct causes that occurred simultaneously. No one knew what was wrong and I only wanted to feel better.

•

Later that night, my skin was so hot someone could've melted cheese on it. I huddled underneath the covers and shook like someone painted my body with ice water. Frigid temperatures gripped the region and our room felt unusually cold. Only a flimsy cotton blanket covered me. At the rate Highgate billed the car insurance company, I deserved a down comforter.

I buzzed my call button and a nurse responded. She gave the aide strict orders to place cold compresses on my shivering body. Cold compresses? I wanted warmth, not cold. This couldn't be true.

"I'm taking off your clothes," the aide said. "Cold compresses will lower your fever."

"Why not wheel me outside and let me lie in the snow."

"This'll make you feel better," the aide said.

By the next day, my fever stayed the same. The rash was now so thick and scaly that drawing blood from my arms was impossible. The nurse tweaked blood samples using the veins in my feet, which hurt so much. That's one memory that remains clear and vivid, just like the gurgling, raspy sound of patients on ventilators.

Dr. Freeman ordered Aveeno baths, an oatmeal mixture that can soothe skin eruptions. An automatic lifting device was the only way to get me into the therapeutic hot tub. Instead of a rehab center, I felt like I was on a conveyor belt. Embarrassed, I sat naked in a wheelchair that was automatically hoisted in the air and then dunked into the water. The entire process took almost an hour. The warmth felt great but the special bath did nothing for the rash or the fever.

More blood and urine tests yielded no clues yet the staff at Highgate still hadn't arranged for a specialist. I wanted to scratch myself into oblivion. Enough car insurance money was available to cover a consultation with a dermatologist or an allergist.

The next morning, thick scaly patches splattered across my face. My eyes were almost shut. A nurse squeezed more blood out of my feet into vials. The pain was excruciating. Once more, the results showed nothing that made sense. I probably had some kind of hospital crud that no one knew how to cure.

The only positive outcome was the discontinuation of Phenobarbital. If nothing else, I trusted my mental outlook would improve. I could wake up without feeling hung over.

The head nurse said I had an outside medical appointment. Fabulous, I would finally see a specialist to end my nightmare. My optimism was short lived because the appointment was at the county hospital for an EEG, a test to measure seizure activity in my brain the results of which said, "Unequivocally abnormal."

"What about the rash?" I asked.

"I don't know. Dr. Freeman didn't mention anything."

"Do something, for crying out loud. I can't stand the itch."

"Let me call the doctor. I don't know what else to do."

By now, I was at an all-time low. I lost faith that Highgate would make me whole again. "Call the doctor for what? Another oatmeal bath?"

Again, I spent most of the next few days in bed. I missed all rehab groups. I slept on and off. The itching nearly drove me insane. I ended up seeing a private doctor outside of the facility who had no idea what caused the rash or the fever but he prescribed a ten-day course of prednisone. Within days I noticed improvement. Years later I discovered that I became allergic to Benadryl, which Highgate administered to treat the rash. Benadryl exacerbated the rash considerably. A dermatologist said for unknown reasons trauma to the body, even childbirth, may cause allergic reactions to drugs, even over-the-counter drugs. I signed myself out of Highgate against medical advice several weeks before my suggested discharge date. I would heal at home with home care.

Chapter Six
Healing at Home Begins

In March, 1994, home therapy started. I was glad to be home although I wasn't sure what awaited me. Would I ever work again? I felt washed up and dried out, like the time I lost my managerial job at a Fortune 500 company way back in 1982, at around the same time I had quit smoking. I healed then and I would have to heal again now.

RIF (reduction in force), downsizing, outsourcing. Those words all mean the same thing. You're fired. A manager uttered those dreaded words to me long ago but the memories of being fired still stirs up fear and anger. Just like now. Why hadn't that driver seen me walking two dogs?

I can't remember the accident but memories of that dreary February morning in 1982 when the department head summoned me to his office still linger. My gut said it wasn't for a friendly chat or a morning bun. With a snarl on his face, the head honcho said I was terminated, just like that. Mr. Cost Cutter said my services were no longer needed. Wipe that caustic smile off your face, I said to myself. You just ruined my life. I was only in my twenties and a few degrees shy of a bachelor's degree. For all my service, I received a modest severance package and pay for unused vacation. The master of my destiny wished me well. I refused to shake Mr. Cost Cutter's outstretched hand. I left the office, ducked into the nearest ladies' room and wept. I cleaned out my office into a tattered paper shopping bag, taking with me memories of Christmas parties, birthday luncheons, and photos of co-workers, a few of whom passed too early. I poked my head into several offices to say goodbye to colleagues. Some could hardly believe I got canned. Everyone was sorry. Yeah, me too. After tears and hugs, I rode the elevator to the lobby, pushed through the revolving doors, and left the building for the last time. Wow, I wasn't coming back to work here. Not ever. There'd be no more lunches at the greasy spoon diner across the street. Just as well. The burgers were grizzly and the coffee weak but it was the joy of eating with co-workers that I'd miss. Holding my shopping bag chock full of memories, I passed by a few clothing stores I had patronized, buying dresses, skirts and slacks that made me look sharp at the office. A lady had to look nice, didn't she? What would my life be without the midtown Manhattan madness? Pushing and shoving was so much a part of my life that I'd miss being jostled by strangers rushing for a train. I'd even long for the stale muffins and the limp lettuce on the BLT sandwiches at the company cafeteria. What now? No more after work drinks with friends, company dinners, viewing the latest movies, or museum openings. I felt dried up and worn out like an old shoe. That's how I felt after the accident.

•

For home therapy, I had to acclimate myself to yet another set of therapists and to an entirely new routine. For someone with short-term memory loss and confusion, another change ruffled me. I always thrived on a schedule to keep me grounded. Second thoughts about leaving Highgate early surfaced. Maybe I should've stayed until my planned discharge date in mid-March. Wait, scrap that thought. At least I was home, sleeping in my own bed and in the company of my dogs and in contact with my friends. Congregate care was so impersonal it robbed me of my dignity. I was glad to bathe and sit on the bowl in private once again.

My readers may wonder why there's no mention of family. My father passed away in 1992. I never had a close relationship with my mother, who died in 2013, or other family members. I wasn't looking for one before or after the accident. I had managed most of my life without family support and would carry on now. Enough said.

•

Here is a side-bar about the home care agency that provided my care. In spring 1993, my job search fanned across Tompkins County. Among other places, I applied as the assistant to the executive director of Visiting Nurse Service. On my resume I left out my social work degree. I played down my experience at previous agencies. I needed a job until I could figure out my career change but the agency rejected me. The director, however, remembered me when I applied for home care services. She promised that I'd receive good care.

Cognitive rehab, which I honestly had never heard of, came via a private contractor named Dori Lester (who once worked at Highgate) since the agency didn't offer this less popular form of rehabilitation therapy. I wondered why I needed cognitive rehab. I held a masters degree, read the *Times* since I was sixteen, and listened to National Public Radio (NPR). Dr. Nick Bella, the psychologist from Highgate said I should pursue it for my own good. I trusted him so I accepted the services, but second thoughts lingered.

By the time outpatient therapy began, I experienced fewer and fewer delusions although I heard an occasional voice. I was never sure what the voices said, however. Almost daily, I was oriented to person, place, and mostly to time, but my brain was shaking up like a box of Cracker Jacks. I was fearful, almost paranoid, when confronted with new situations. Strangers made me uncomfortable. I had trouble retrieving words from simple conversations. My thoughts and speech pulled me in different directions, sometimes making me feel stretched like salt water taffy. I couldn't center myself anymore. Some of these issues still linger many years later. Only two wet noses, Judy and Maxine, gave me a reason to get up. I was crushed that I couldn't jog with them anymore. At least they didn't end up in a shelter and I wasn't in a group home.

•

The Visiting Nurse Service dispatched a nurse, a rather pleasant young woman, to see me shortly after discharge named Marta Kaminski. I was on decreasing doses of prednisone at the time for the rash, which improved daily. There was no more fever. The nurse asked if I knew how to take the medication. I said I did. Marta asked me a few times to make sure. The nurse then posted a medication schedule on my refrigerator for extra assurance. Several visits later, Marta stopped coming. My health had been excellent prior to the accident and my condition was labeled as chronic but stable. The nurse left the door open in case I needed her. That was fine with me.

•

Every time a visiting therapist knocked at the front door my two dogs yapped in unison. Once a therapist walked in, the dogs sniffed at the stranger's feet then settled down for yet another nap. With the occupational and physical therapists, I followed exercises to rebuild my stamina, walking, and balance as well as activities of daily living. Their twice weekly visits lasted about forty-five minutes, give or take on my fatigue level. Like many patients who sustained a TBI, I faced a lot of fatigue. The exercises often wore me out. I sometimes asked the therapist to end the session early. I was just too tired to continue.

The cognitive therapist, Dori Lester, worked on my memory because in the brief time I had been home, I set a small fire, locked the dogs out in a rainstorm, and misplaced several important documents. In addition, I blistered my hands because I didn't always remember to use mitts when removing hot plates from the oven. I filled up the bathtub then forgot to take a bath. I found a shoe in the freezer and a new plate in the trash. If I was going to survive on my own, my memory had to improve. Otherwise, I might be cited as a danger to myself or to others. That could land me in the psych ward against my will. I couldn't let that happen.

•

Bit by bit, I slowly progressed but nothing was ever the same. My memory improved but large holes went unfilled. Using a four-pronged cane, I walked with difficulty, losing my balance easily. Thankfully, I never broke any bones. I tired easily. How different from the days when I ran several miles in the morning then worked all day. Compromised neurologically as well as from multiple breaks, my left hand felt weak and painful. Still, I persevered each day. There was no turning back.

•

Not long after home therapy began, I made an appointment with the same neurologist who evaluated me at Highgate—Dr. John Cook. He shared an office with the only other neurologist in the county. Keeping with standard medical tradition, the doctor was late, very late. Unlike other medical offices, the waiting area was empty except for me. The decor was drab like a medieval convent. Family oriented magazines were outdated, the framed pictures were dowdy, and the furniture looked like it came from Good Will. Where was a juicy issue of *People*?

After a while, I asked the receptionist, "Will the wait be much longer?"

The receptionist barely lifted her shoulders and said, "He's busy." I just grunted.

A frustrating wait ended when the doctor finally called my name. A skinny man with dirty blond hair and horn-rimmed glasses, Dr. Cook appeared to be in his early to mid-thirties. On the way to his office, he never once turned around to greet me. Even though we had met earlier, I don't remember anything about him. If my mind had been in full swing, surely, I would've remembered this ice-cold man.

Dr. Cook spoke to me like a naughty child, ordering me to an exam room. Arms firmly folded across his upper chest, he said, "Lift both legs as fast as you can."

Due to my left-sided weakness I could only move so fast. I thought he was pushy instead of sympathetic. Or maybe that's how he motivated people to improve and I was resistant.

He sounded as if he was scolding a high school football team. "Come on, do better."

I felt like asking him to show some compassion.

He shifted to my left hand. "Squeeze your fingers and make a fist." I tried but failed. "Did you hear me?"

Yes, doctor, I'm not deaf. "My hand still hurts. It was broken in the accident."

Dr. Cook let go of a loud sucking sound, as if annoyed. I sensed my relationship with him would be adversarial, like the mood between hospitals and insurance companies. I left with nothing more than an appointment to return in two months. I wondered why I should.

•

Sessions with Dori Lester the cognitive therapist dumped a new load of frustration into my lap. Similar to other brain damaged people, I assumed my intellectual abilities were more intact than they were. I resisted the idea I needed help. Memory was always one of my strong points. I rarely wrote down dates, addresses or phone numbers. Instead, my brain absorbed loads of details and stored them until needed. I sailed through statistics with an A not because I understood the complex concepts, but rather I memorized dozens of formulas, most of which meant nothing to me. The accident introduced sudden changes I had no choice but to cope with. I had to write down everything. There were notes scattered all over the house, reminding me to call certain people, to feed the dogs, or to take out the trash. Mostly it worked but sometimes I forgot to jot down an important task.

•

Home therapy continued each week but I soon felt detached from my team. No one it seemed wanted to mention the word "disability." The serious accident left me with permanent lifelong injuries. How could it not? There was damage to my brain that included swelling and bleeding. My therapy team had a version of making me whole but I couldn't return to pre-accident state, no matter how hard I tried. I wanted to improve my mobility skills so I could walk further than around the house without having to sit down. My legs just wouldn't cooperate. I wanted to toss a Frisbee at Judy my dog with my left hand but it always felt limp and flaccid. My grasp wasn't coming back. Details that once wedged themselves inside my head now quickly faded. Most of all, I was petrified the home therapy team would send me back to work. I cringed at the idea of packing boxes and typing labels again. Maybe if I held a thrilling career I would've been more motivated in-home therapy.

I also fretted about living independently on the monthly pittance from Social Security. They approved my disability application right away and my benefits began in August 1994. Approval for Social Security relieved me. At least I'd have an income again, albeit small. On the other hand, did this mean I was really disabled? Would I ever rejoin the workforce? I had always worked and supported myself, even if I lived from one paycheck to the next. What would happen to me since I started to collect Social Security at such a young age? There would be no pension to supplement my meager income. Overwhelmed, I couldn't think about what the future held for me. I dreaded getting out of bed.

On top of that, the accident temporarily swept away my earlier writing aspirations. Control over my life seemed to whittle away. I was in a deep funk and terrified of the future.

Chapter Seven
Settling the Case

A huge stack of unread magazines wanted my attention but reading them all was out of the question. I couldn't digest what I read. Memory restoration was still a work in progress and my vision was uncooperative. I felt like shredding *Mother Jones* and the other issues because they presented such a challenge to me. For the heck of it, I tried a *New York Times* crossword puzzle and was stumped by the word apple. I thought it meant apply. Instead, I watched television and slept in between therapy sessions. Snuggling up with Judy and Maxine always made me feel better, even if I sometimes forgot to feed them. They never complained.

Every now and then, I received a call or a visit from a friend. Connections were just warming up before the accident so I only had a few local friends. I appreciated the occasional visits but most people moved on with their lives. Few had time for me anymore. Friends from New York City visited but the commute between the Ithaca area and the city was at least five hours. City friends didn't have cars and the bus ride took at least seven hours so I was alone a lot. That was hard to accept. Ever since kindergarten, an active social network surrounded me.

My largely solitary life served another purpose. It shielded me from embarrassment. There were so many things I couldn't remember or failed to understand. Judy and Maxine were my only salvation. To them, I was still top dog no matter what or who I forgot.

A lawyer, Kevin Bedi, pursued damages against the driver and his insurance carrier. Serious injury cases call for legal representation. He warned me not to expect a large settlement because the driver carried limited liability insurance.

"Suing people personally is hard. Most hide assets when something like this happens," Kevin said. "I doubt this guy has much. He works as a maintenance man."

Besides the driver's lack of insurance, I had no eye witnesses.

New to the arena of litigation, I had no idea what to expect. "What're you saying?"

"You probably won't get more than $50,000, no matter how much I scream at the insurance company. Policy limits apply."

And, of course, the lawyer got a generous third for not much more than making a few calls.

Since I got bounced around like luggage on an airport conveyor belt, I expected the settlement would be larger. I heard about lawsuits where minimally injured people collected big bucks. "If a truck from a big company hit you, I'd be able to work out a much larger settlement," Bedi said. "The driver had $50,000 in liability insurance and you carried $75,000. Your insurance company has to pay the difference." He of course got a third.

I expected the insurance company to throw up roadblocks. The insurance giant seemed overly eager to hold onto their money. "Won't they be thrilled?"

"Too bad." My lawyer winked. "Leave it up to me, but remember things takes time."

For as long as I could recall, I slogged along in low paying jobs and never had more than a few hundred dollars in the bank. I cut coupons, watched for sales, and picked out clothes in thrift shops in ritzy neighborhoods. My dad worked in a factory and his wages barely kept us housed in a crappy apartment. Lunch was sometimes sliced bread and canned pineapple.

I expected or hoped for more than the amount Bedi quoted me. Hospitalized for almost two months I would be hobbled with lifelong injuries. Such was life and I had to live with the settlement. Take it or leave it.

•

I visited Rosie, my roommate at Highgate, a few weeks after I left. A friend drove me to the rehab center. I thought I'd be antsy going back to the rehab center but I wasn't. I looked for the muscle man who threatened to make me eat but he wasn't around. A few staff members remembered me and asked how I was. Smiling, I said fine, thank you.

I found Rosie seated upright in a chair. I bent down and hugged her. "I missed you." That I meant.

"Ready to go home now." Rosie's speech remained slurred.

Over the past few weeks, Rosie graduated from a wheelchair to a walker. "Seems like you're making good progress," I said, proud of my friend's accomplishments. For a long time, Rosie could not walk at all.

"Maybe so," she said. "Maybe so."

In spite of garbled words and choppy sentences, I understood Rosie. As we talked, though, her thoughts suddenly faded away. She stared idly into space. To draw her back into the conversation, I called out her name once or twice. Like many head injured patients, including me, Rosie frequently changed the subject and repeated herself.

"Ready to go. Dinner time soon."

"What about discharge?" I asked.

She dropped her head and said, "Not yet."

I sensed how much she ached to go home and I promised to visit her again soon if I could get a ride. I still hadn't returned to driving. I felt fortunate to be home and not in a congregate care facility.

•

I refused to become a TV addict yet I needed another way to occupy myself now that I was home all the time. Returning to social work wasn't possible due to memory loss, fatigue, and confusion. My left hand was badly damaged so typing for a living, as much as I dreaded the thought, would've been out of the question. I still use only two fingers on my left hand when behind the computer.

One day, friends drove me to the Carousel Mall in Syracuse, about an hour north of Ithaca. On a whim, I bought a jigsaw puzzle. Completing the 1,000-piece puzzle took me weeks but I enjoyed it. In an odd way, the puzzle challenged my feeble memory. Jigsaw puzzles were also a cheap form of entertainment. After completing the puzzle, I felt a sense of accomplishment. On my return trip to the Syracuse mall, I stocked up on more puzzles.

Chilly weather smothered much of upstate NY that winter. All the windows in the house were sealed shut as they had been since September. So were the doors. Not until late May or early June did it warm enough to let in the fresh air.

I sat in the living room, excited as I pieced together a new puzzle. For a brief time, I felt content. My dogs rested comfortably nearby. Suddenly, the inside living room door blew open and there was a weird tingling sensation, as if someone else was in the room. I grabbed my cane to inspect the outside door, which remained closed. This couldn't be a Shirley MacLaine episode of *Out on a Limb* so I tried to logically explain why the inside door suddenly popped open when this never happened before. My dogs jumped up and stared at the open door with tails curled between their legs. Nothing made sense so I returned to the couch and resumed working on the puzzle. I was a bit scared but it's not like I could run away. Then, my heart bounced around like a ball on full court press. The lid to my Snausages dog treat jar on the kitchen counter opened and it played its greeting, "Snausages, Snausages." I had saved enough coupons from the popular dog snack to qualify for a free canister that I still have. Every time the top was lifted, the greeting played. It was impossible, just impossible, for the lid to lift on its own. With jittery knees, I approached the kitchen, not sure who or what I would find. Nothing was there but the open canister repeating "Snausages" over and over until I put the lid down. OK, that was it.

I'd heard stories of visitors from the beyond making contact through all kinds of ways, even with our pets. Instead of freaking out, I was convinced that my late father who died in 1992 from lung cancer, was trying to let me know I'd find my way. Why my father? I don't know but I just felt that way. My dad had Alzheimer's and a strong connection to his dog. He would've loved the Snausages canister had he been alive. Although I cannot prove my dad paid me a visit that day in 1994, there is no doubt in my brain damaged mind that I witnessed an unexplained event. Some might say my mind played tricks. The Snausages canister opened by itself, as did the living room door, which had been securely closed. Some things in life have no logical explanations. I experienced one that day.

·

In late spring, I had another appointment with Dr. Cook the neurologist. I would rather have watched the A-Team instead. Like the last time, he kept me waiting. I asked the receptionist, who had an ego the size of a cannon, why such a wait. She barely glanced at me and said, "He's busy."

"There's no one else here," I said.

"I said he was busy." His receptionist spoke to me like I was a naughty kindergarten child.

Another fifteen minutes passed before the doctor appeared. He nodded at me then paraded down the hall to his office. I resented the lack of healthcare choices in rural areas. I considered the idea of seeing his partner, but I presumed he was as much of a creep as he was.

Dr. Cook performed no physical examination except to check the grasp on my left hand. The swelling had subsided, but I remained unable to make a tight fist. I winced when bending my fingers.

"How's your eyesight? Still have double vision?" he asked.

"I've been seeing Dr. Kennedy for vision therapy. Seems to help."

"You're seeing *him*?" Obviously he disapproved, as if I cared. "Come back in two months."

For this I waited half an hour? He got paid for it too. I needed that kind of job.

•

Eventually, Dr. Bella succeeded where I failed and assembled a team meeting of my outpatient therapists to talk about my progress, where I was headed, and what other steps, if any, they should take for my care.

In writing this book, I checked one of the home therapist's notes. "Ongoing communication between all team members will be sought." That never happened. She got paid well for work not always accomplished.

Dr. Bella took the lead and explained the nature of head trauma. He summarized my case and the injuries I sustained. The meeting went along smoothly until the physical therapist faced the others and said, "I think she should look for a little part-time job or something and maybe do filing or stuff envelopes." She acted as if I didn't exist yet I was almost forty years old with a masters degree.

I felt invisible and no, I didn't want a little part-time job filing. I wasn't sure what I could do, but no matter what happened I refused to accept menial work ever again. Tears rolled down my cheeks as I worked to keep my cool.

"You speak about me as if I don't exist when I'm sitting right here," I said.

Dr. Bella sensed the physical therapist's suggestion was inappropriate and impractical. He handed me a tissue and confronted her.

"That's not a good idea," Dr. Bella said. He explained why considering I had lingering problems with memory, ambulation, and a compromised left hand.

"Please address me directly," I said, "and don't talk as if I don't exist."

Dr. Bella forged ahead. "Let's wrap things up."

I never saw the purpose in the group meeting. Nothing useful ever came of it. Each therapist had their agenda but it wasn't my agenda. They rarely talked to each other or to my physicians, even though I signed consent forms to do so. Maybe I wasn't the easiest patient to work with either. I had been fiercely independent and now I was in a deep funk. Nothing was the same nor would it be. I continued with home therapy until the fall. I occasionally had private therapy sessions with Dr. Bella. And I moved forward in a very uncertain world.

•

That summer, I accepted the $50,000 settlement, minus a generous cut for my lawyer, from the driver's insurance company, Metropolitan Life. As Mr. Bedi handed me the check, he said, "I'm sorry I couldn't get more."

"Yeah, me too."

Once I signed forms releasing the driver from culpability, Mr. Bedi placed a check for $33,000 in to my sweaty, trembling hand. That was the most money I had in my entire life. Maybe it'd be the most I would ever have. The only other large check made out to me was for $12,500, the proceeds of a student loan to finish social work school. NYU deducted two thirds for tuition and left me the rest. My heart pounded when I folded the $33,000 check and slid it inside my wallet. For just a moment, I struck gold but, too bad, gold didn't last.

"Wait," my lawyer said, "The insurance company owes you money, but they're giving me a hard time."

Paranoid with a check that large in my wallet, I was convinced some crook would snatch it from me. I had no immediate plans to spend it. I would finally have a savings account with more than a few hundred dollars in it.

I bought a new car with cash, well not cash, but a check. I couldn't drive my old car, which was a stick shift. It was just too confusing for me. I paid off some bills, donated some to charity, and put the rest away for a rainy day. Over the years, I had too many rainy days and there wasn't much left.

One day, at Dr. Bella's behest, I accepted information about monthly meetings of the support group for brain injured patients. Initially, I balked at the idea of going, convinced it wasn't for me. I wouldn't have anything to say. Just the opposite happened. I fit right in.

Most people were involved in car accidents, but a construction worker slipped off a roof and fractured his skull. Some had trouble speaking, a few used wheelchairs, and one man was opinionated and obnoxious. Then there was Linda, who was profoundly disabled from a near fatal car accident many years ago. Linda lived in a nearby group home.

Attending just a few of these meetings convinced me never to see myself as a victim, particularly because of Linda who was profoundly impaired. Barely able to speak, she was confined to a wheel chair, wore adult diapers and had to be fed. From the group leader, I found out family hardly visited. I started to visit her about once a week. Maybe the helper in me was revived. Communication was difficult but Linda's eyes said she recognized me. I just sat with her and talked. Sometimes, I read from a book or magazine. I didn't know what else to do once she was hospitalized. I wasn't sure for what reason but I visited her. A few months later I made plans to leave the area. I brought Linda a bouquet of flowers and told her why my visits would end. I hugged her goodbye. There were tears in both our eyes. Linda came into my life for a brief moment to teach me a lesson about self-pity. I took a whacking in the car accident. My injuries were significant but compared to Linda, I ended up very fortunate. She remained dependent on others for the rest of her life. At least I left congregate care. She never did.

Chapter Eight
Moving Right Along

In November, Dr. Bella said I should undergo a neuropsychological evaluation, a lengthy test to gauge how my cognitive skills had improved, if at all, since the accident.

The marathon test covers a wide range of skills, such as language, speech, memory and learning, attention and concentration, spatial and perceptual processing, and emotional functioning. I took it in two three-hour sessions. Among the findings were:

- Ms. White demonstrated a decline on measures of general intellectual functioning from her expected pre-morbid levels.
- Her arithmetic achievement was significantly poorer than her reading and spelling skills.
- Ms. White showed difficulty in the speed which she shifted between sets when presented with a timed task.
- Ms. White demonstrated some problems in generating novel concepts. She also had difficulty in generalizing a principle to new stimulus configurations, even after she has demonstrated evidence that she had mastered the principle.
- Ms. White demonstrated significant difficulties in memory and learning.
- Ms. White was weak and slow bilaterally.
- Ms. White demonstrated good retention of old vocabulary.

The results made me feel like I had sponge cake upstairs for brains. Sidetracked by the results, I decided to look at the brighter side. My vocabulary skills were good so I took that as a sign to keep writing. I had nothing to lose by moving forward.

•

In late March 1995, a colleague suggested I seek a second neurological opinion. She recommended Dr. Allen Durand in Syracuse. Fabulous idea. I wasn't satisfied with Dr. Cook and saw no reason for continued visits to his office.

I called Dr. Durand right away for an appointment. His secretary said the doctor spoke with all new patients. The next day, Dr. Durand returned my call, sounding pleasant and upbeat at 7:15 a.m. I was barely awake when he asked, "Why do you want to see a neurologist?"

His offbeat manners, plus the early hour, left me momentarily speechless. "I...I...was hit by a van and I have a head injury."

"What kind?"

"A contusion to the frontal lobe."

"I limit my practice to patients with multiple sclerosis, but I'll see you. Call my secretary and tell her I said it's OK."

Two weeks later, a friend drove me to Syracuse. I sat in Dr. Durand's packed waiting room. Ten to fifteen minutes passed and he called me into his office. Even then, he apologized for the wait. I already felt good about him.

Like a host welcoming a guest into his home, Dr. Durand escorted me into an exam room. Two medical students followed. "Is it OK if they stay?" he asked.

Having worked for years in a large medical center, I understood that taking part in physical exams was crucial to their education. "Sure, I don't mind."

Dr. Durand and the two students checked me for everything. Besides a physical exam, Dr. Durand performed extensive mental testing as well. His notes showed my thought processes were slowed and it took me a long time to get accurate answers about who is the president, vice president, and so on.

Unlike Dr. Cook who saw me every two months and basically said nothing, Dr. Durand ordered a series of MRI films. Sometimes damage not visible on a CT scan appears on the more advanced MRI he said.

Five days later I learned the results. "Subtle posterior focus of hemosiderin... as well as mild ventriculomegaly... and the cavum septi pellucidi are compatible with injury." I wished the MRI films had been taken at the time of my injury or during the course of home therapy. Maybe the home therapists would've seen me as lazy or uninterested. At that point, it no longer mattered.

"Do I need to come back?" If I needed a neurologist, it would be Dr. Durand and surely not Dr. Cook.

"No reason to." Dr. Durand hugged me. "Sorry I can't do more."

"Dr. Cook has me see him every two months."

Dr. Durand grabbed both my hands and said, "He's wasting your insurance company's money and your time." At least it wasn't my own money.

That was the last of Dr. Cook. I never returned to his office.

•

To keep in shape, I took out a pool membership at a local hotel. The insurance compant paid my bill because it was an extension of physical therapy. Jogging was no longer a possibility so I switched to water therapy. There was virtually no chance for injury unless I drowned. That was unlikely since the pool was four feet at its deepest part. I wore a weight belt to swim because my legs and arms didn't cooperate the way they once did. After one or two attempts, I got the hang of swimming and enjoyed my new exercise. A sauna in the women's dressing room relaxed me after a swim. I also enjoyed getting out of the house.

•

When springtime arrived in 1995, tiny green buds blossomed on the trees. The sugary sweet smells of our lilac bushes tickled my nose. Vestiges of the frigid winter were gone, at least for another season.

One day as I sat on the small scrap of a front porch, I thought about getting out more often. I called my family physician, Dr. Edward Parker, and asked him to support my request for a motorized scooter. Friends often helped out by driving me to appointments but I wanted to become independent. My left hand and wrist were compromised so there would be limits to my pushing a wheelchair. A motorized scooter would allow me greater freedom. I still grumbled about living in the cold, but I needed wheels for independence.

A neighbor drove me to Syracuse for me to check out a medical supply company. There were none nearby. I settled on a scooter with a price tag of $4,000, average for motorized scooters to use outside. The final tab also included a portable ramp to get the scooter in and out of the house.

A few days later a claims adjuster from the insurance company called. "We will not approve your request for a scooter."

"Why not?" I asked.

"It's too expensive," the adjuster said.

"Less costly scooters are for indoor use. I need one for outdoors."

"I'll call you back," he said.

The adjuster said to expect a visit from a case manager. "I've been out of Highgate for over a year. Why now a case manager?"

"Please cooperate. We want to make sure you get the right equipment."

Oh please. Similar to insurance companies everywhere, mine was tight fisted. Power operated vehicles are expensive yet they allow disabled people to live as independently as possible. I was incensed the insurance company tried to deny me independence.

·

At the end of a lengthy examination, a nurse hired by the insurance company said, "I've reviewed your records from the various hospitals, home therapy, and from Dr. Parker." She jotted down notes. "You meet at least three of the criteria five needed for a scooter."

Snag on you. The insurance company probably hired the nurse to deny my request. In her final report, she noted the insurance company should be prepared to spend the remainder of the policy, about another $25,000.

Perhaps as a way to flex their corporate muscle, the insurance company insisted I deal with a supplier they located about ninety minutes away in Binghamton. In the end, this scooter cost a mere $200 less than the one I originally picked out in Syracuse. Despite the insurance company's tightwad approach to save a few bucks, they ended up paying $2,357.79 for the nurse's evaluation in addition to the scooter. Finally, I got my hot wheels and I billed them for gas to make the trip.

Chapter Nine
Managed Care Blues

The insurance vipers struck again. Dated October 2, 1995, a letter from Claims Adjustors (CA), a managed care company, arrived that sidetracked me from a slow but steady recovery. At the behest of the auto insurance company, CA instructed me to appear at the office of Dr. Richard Montini, a psychologist, on November 7 for "an independent medical examination." I suspected they wanted a neuro-psych exam, which I had already taken almost one year ago. I doubt much had changed since then. I noticed the location and balked. Dr. Montini's Rochester office was nearly three hours away. My insurance nightmare was about to unfold.

After fuming then I cried. Once I regained a shred of self-control, I called Kevin Bedi, my lawyer. Fortunately, he was available.

"Calm down," Kevin said. "Tell me everything."

I read the letter, word for word. "Who is CA?" I asked. "Never heard of these people."

"A managed care company, stooges for the insurance company."

"I'm not part of managed care," I said.

"I'll look into it and call you back."

The auto insurance company hired CA to determine if I was still disabled. Several months earlier, the insurance company paid to have me evaluated for a motorized scooter. That exam showed a permanent, lifelong disability. A miracle hadn't occurred in such a short time.

"Dr. Montini isn't a physician," I said. "How can he make a medical determination?"

"This is a neuro-psych exam and I asked them to use someone local. I reminded them you can't legally drive yet."

"Why Dr. Montini, he's not even close to where I live?"

"That's the insurance's boy and gives them results they want. I'll draft a letter asking for a change of venue. Meanwhile, try and relax."

I called Dr. Bella for an appointment the following day. I was about to melt from the pressure.

As soon as I entered Dr. Bella's office, I said, "The insurance company wants me to see Dr. Montini for an independent medical exam." I fell into a chair without taking off my coat.

Dr. Bella groaned. "This is off the record."

"I probably won't remember anyway." We laughed for a second or two.

"The insurance company forces head injured people to see Montini. Unless they're almost brain dead, Montini says everything is fine. They use him as a way to cut benefits. I've testified in court against him many times."

"They've already paid over $75,000 in medical bills. I only have about $25,000 left. Why now?"

"The insurance company is showing you they're in charge."

"Why can't you do the test?" I asked. "You did the last one."

"My palms aren't greased by the insurance industry."

I stared out the window.

The insurance company's heavy hand tightened the noose. A letter dated October 17 said, "Enclosed is a new medical authorization. Please sign it and return it in the enclosed envelope provided. Please return it as soon as possible so we can continue to process your claim in an efficient manner."

What lies. The insurance company had stalled and took weeks to pay claims while providers pressed me for payment, threatening litigation. Again, I called Kevin and told him about the latest missive.

"They want me to sign another medical authorization," I said.

"Add a disclaimer that says this authorization is only for records related to the motor vehicle accident of January 6, 1994. Otherwise, they'll look through your past history to explain your current problems."

"Nothing was wrong with my brain before the accident," I said, although some might argue that. "The insurance company isn't fair."

Following Kevin's orders, I popped my response in the mail. A few days later, another letter arrived. Either the insurance company hadn't received Kevin's letter asking for a change of venue or they ignored it. This letter said, "You have an appointment for an examination by Dr. Montini scheduled for November 7, 1995. In order for him to do as thorough examination as possible, he is going to have to obtain as much of your history, including medical, employment, and educational information, as he can. The more information he can obtain, the better he can evaluate your present psychological and medical status."

Instead of foaming at the mouth, I reached Kevin and read the letter. "This guy can't evaluate my medical status."

"I'll get the insurance company on the phone and see what's going on," he said.

Over the next several weeks, Kevin tried to reason with the insurance company. At least a dozen licensed psychologists practiced in the Ithaca area and could have administered the neuro-psych exam. Again, he reminded the insurance company I couldn't legally drive yet. The insurance company insisted only a board-certified neuropsychologist could administer the exam and Dr. Montini was only one of three such psychologists in the entire state of New York. I found that hard to believe. Thousands of psychologists were licensed in New York State.

In a follow-up visit with Dr. Bella, I told him what the insurance company had said.

"Rubbish," Dr. Bella said. "All kinds of psychological boards exist that I can join if I paid the annual dues. A state license is what counts. The obscure board that Montini belongs to means nothing. The insurance company is stretching it for their advantage."

"Will they cut off my benefits?"

"That'd be foolish," Dr. Bella said, "since he's not a medical doctor."

Not long after I got home, I listened to the answering machine. Kevin had called. His message said, "CA wants to send Dr. Montini to your house to conduct the exam."

That's an invasion of my privacy, I said to myself, and I don't want that charlatan in my house.

One more time, Kevin asked CA to have the test administered locally and the insurance giant balked. On November 27, I received yet another letter from CA. "This is to confirm your independent medical examination requested by the insurance company has been rescheduled to December 29, 1995 at 9:00 a.m."

Evidently the insurance company or CA paid no attention to Kevin's letters or phone calls. He called the next morning. "The test is off for now, but they'll be back."

"I'm sure they will," I said.

The insurance company's scare tactics dampened my holiday spirit. Two days after a gloomy Christmas, I watched a movie. The crackle of burning wood warmed the house. Both dogs rested nearby. The phone rang and I jumped up to answer it. Dr. Montini called to remind me I was due in his office.

"Dr. Montini, I can't drive and have no way of getting to your office," I said. "What do you want me to do?"

"No one told me that," Montini said, "I'll have to tell the insurance company."

"Quit hassling me," I said, hanging up the phone. I went to bed instead of watching the end of the movie.

On New Year's Eve, a damp, gloomy day, the mailman knocked on the door. A certified letter needed my signature. Not knowing it was from the insurance company, I signed the form. The envelope contained a claim denial that said, "All no-fault benefits are denied, effective immediately, due to your non-cooperation and failure to submit to an independent medical examination by Dr. Montini, scheduled for December 29, 1995." What to do first? Cry, scream, or torch the local insurance company building? The corporate sleaze made me miserable.

On January 9, 1996, Kevin fired off a letter to a supervisor at the insurance company, stressing the illegality of denying medical benefits based on a psychologist's say so. Part of his letter also said, "The exam appears wholly unnecessary." He questioned Dr. Montini's credentials, referring to them as "suspect."

Several days later, Kevin received the insurance company's reply. "I am perplexed at the accusatory and threatening tone of your letter. Our denial was issued based on the grounds that your client failed to keep the appointment with Dr. Montini which she knew about weeks in advance." Once more, the insurance company refused to acknowledge I had no way of reaching Dr. Montini's office. Well, friends could've driven me but I refused to ask. Why make it easy for the insurance giant?

The letter ended with, "I understand that Debra is willing to submit to an independent medical examination. We are, therefore, revoking the denial of December 28, 1995. We want the examination rescheduled immediately. Failure to attend this examination will greatly jeopardize all future no-fault benefits." The insurance company's use of the word "immediately" made me feel like a two-bit cheater. Did a lengthy hospital stay and a year of home therapy with substantial medical records prove I had been seriously injured?

On February 2, 1996 Kevin sent the insurance company yet another letter questioning the insurance company's repeated demand that Dr. Montini conduct the exam. "The selection of examiner is also questionable. We have discussed that Dr. Montini, rightly or wrongly, has a reputation in the medical and insurance community for producing results which are highly favorable to the insurance carriers who sponsor his examinations. I note the insurance company has rejected my repeated requests to select any one of a number of qualified examiners other than Dr. Montini. The insurance company's insistence upon Dr. Montini appears biased toward a particular result." I doubted the corporate giant would take this lying down.

A letter dated February 8, 1996, scheduled an appointment with Dr. Montini on February 23 and 24. Also included was an unlikely list of documents Montini needed for the exam.

- All medical records prior to 1/6/94 from all primary care physicians.
- High school grade transcripts and standardized test results.
- College transcripts.
- Police accident report from 1/6/94.
- Acute hospital records including: ED notes from 1/6/94, CT or MRI reports, and discharge summaries by all professionals.
- All OB/GYN records.
- All records from Dr. Bella including private practice and Highgate records.
- All pharmacy records for two years prior to 1/6/94 up to present date.

A subsequent letter to Kevin, dated February 13, 1996, reiterated the insurance company's choice of Dr. Montini as the examiner. The letter ended with, "Your letter contains an extremely adversarial tone. If this is your intent, I regret it, it is not mine. We simply wish to have an independent exam completed for the reasons previously stated." At least they finally stopped referring to the test as a medical exam. Those scrooges had nerve accusing Kevin of being adversarial.

I remained unyielding about access to my OB/GYN records. The status of my reproductive organs wasn't connected to my brain injury.

Moreover, I graduated from high school in 1972; it was now 1996. My high school records would serve no useful purpose at this point. They would find out I failed religion in junior year and was mischievous. I got sent to the principal's office for hiding in the chapel in freshman year when I cut algebra. Since the insurance company pressed me, I signed a release form for those records, without saying the school went belly up. Let them waste time and money trying to secure copies of records probably buried inside some distant warehouse.

No pharmacy records for the two years prior to January 6, 1994 existed. Even if I had taken prescription medication, I refused to share that knowledge with the insurance company. It had no relationship to the car accident.

I signed for my college records but omitted the year I graduated or from what school. Let them figure it out.

On February 14, Kevin wrote to CA about their request. "Such records are not only outside Dr. Montini's known expertise, they also have no conceivable relevance to assessment of the claimant's head injury. The demands for pharmacy records prior to January 6, 1994 up to present date are similarly overbroad. The claimant will require proof of Dr. Montini's expertise to review the demanded medical records and of their relevance to her examination before she will produce any such records." Finally, the insurance company relented on the medical records, except those related to the accident. I had no issue with that.

For the test, the insurance company hired car service to escort me to and from Dr. Montini's office in Syracuse, which the insurance company rented just for the exam. At least they accepted I was unable to drive.

As the exam neared, anxiety shrouded me. Simple tasks like cooking became problematic. Numerous times, I forgot to add water to a pot and scorched a batch of green beans, broccoli, and asparagus. I tried to slice a tomato for a salad and ended up nearly cutting off the tip of my finger instead. I had trouble sleeping. My dogs kept me company as I sat in the living room, fretting about the insurance company.

"Should be glad you're dogs," I said, as they slobbered on me.

I watched them fall asleep. I then joined them and let the worries of my world slip away.

Around noon on February 23, a man driving a shabby limousine showed up at my doorstep. I asked the driver how much his company charged by the hour. "Don't worry, doll. The insurance people are taking care of the bill." Although I didn't have a paper and pen, I estimated the round-trip transportation to be well over $2,000. That plus Dr. Montini's hotel and office rental would probably add another $3,500 to $4,000 to the bill. In contrast, Dr. Bella performed the first exam for about $1,400. Did the insurance company honestly expect me to believe this test was for my own benefit? Eat crow, insurance idiots.

Dressed in a sharp, three-piece suit, starched cotton button down shirt, and shiny wing tips, Dr. Montini looked more like a banker than a psychologist. Surprisingly, his rental office smelled like stale socks.

After exactly two hours, I halted the test. "I'm tired. I can't do anymore," I said, yawning as if I hadn't slept in days. I refused to budge even an inch. I intended to make this process as infuriating for the insurance company as they made it for me.

Dr. Montini frowned. "You sure?"

I got up and met the limo driver outside. And off we went. I thought about returning with air freshener.

I ended up taking an extra session to complete the test. I could've handled two sessions, but I wanted to squander the insurance company's money. I didn't care if Dr. Montini returned for an unplanned session.

Test results weren't made available until June. Even then, I pestered the insurance company several times to get the report. As expected, Dr. Montini claimed I intentionally manipulated the test. He claimed ignorance as to why. Some test takers invented brain damage as a way to win larger settlements or to obtain further medical benefits. I had already settled with the insurance company in 1994. In 1996, I wasn't trying to pry more medical benefits from them. At the time of the test, I was no longer in therapy, except for occasional visits with Dr. Bella. I still don't know what purpose this mind-boggling ordeal served. Is it any wonder why companies sometimes lose money?

For Dr. Montini's last dig at his rival Dr. Bella, he said, "It may be advisable for her to have a new mental health specialist take a fresh look at her current status." Stuff it, Montini. I liked, trusted, and respected Dr. Bella, which was more than I could say about that swine shrink. He disgraced his fine profession.

I never let go of my disdain for the insurance company or the blood sucking insurance industry in general. Jerking people around to enhance their bottom line is the only game they know. And they want us to believe they care about the policyholder? By the way, I kept copies of all the correspondence related to my accident.

Chapter Ten
My New Life as a Volunteer in Arizona

In early summer of 1996, I left the Finger Lakes region to escape biting cold, blustery winds, and snow. Oh, that snow. Savage winter storms gripped the region and I didn't like the challenges that followed. First, I had to shovel a path from the house into the yard so my dogs could go out. Dealing with my car was next. If the storm brought along an icy cold wave, I prayed the car would start. Sometimes it did, sometimes it did not. I paid an annual membership to the Automobile Association of America otherwise known as AAA, a most worthy cause. AAA, assuming weather conditions were not dangerous, would send out a driver to jump start my car. If my car started, and most times it did, I turned on the heat as soon as the engine warmed up. That often took time but with heat blasting from inside, the ice melted off the windows much quicker than I could chop it off. There was also the backbreaking task to dig the driveway clear of snow. I hoped and prayed as I drove to work that I wouldn't skid off the road. Driving on slick, icy roads was treacherous as well as scary. Winter time was the scene of numerous fender benders as well as serious car accidents. Dressing in the winter was time consuming because I had to don boots, gloves, sweaters, scarves, gloves, hats, and a coat. Sometimes, that wasn't enough to shield myself from the harsh cold that smacked me in the face as soon as I opened the front door.

After the accident, I no longer drove in the winter. Friends pitched in and escorted me to doctor's appointments, to shop for groceries, or just to get out of the house. I sometimes used a van service twice a week made available by the county. I didn't want to be shut inside.

Now that I felt recovered enough from the accident and sick of drawn out, cold, and snowy winters, I packed up my belongings, my two dogs, and said farewell to central New York. Because of mobility issues, I needed a warmer climate without a lot of precipitation. I tried Florida for a few months but that didn't work out so I moved to Phoenix in 1997. I never left and don't plan to either. At this stage in life, I'm too old to start all over. This is home, even though summers can be sweltering and long. I'll sizzle here before I ever return to a frigid climate.

After my beloved Maxine died in 2001, Judy needed a new companion. I visited the county animal shelter. Hundreds of cast-off mixes and purebreds yapped for attention. Every cage was occupied with unwanted dogs. Their eyes melted my heart, pleading for love and attention. I could only take one. Who would it be?

Luke wasn't on my list. Other dogs had more spunk. A fat black mix with a cute wiggle grabbed my attention but an employee steered me toward Luke, a large curly-haired terrier mix with sad eyes and light brown fur. What shelter dog doesn't have sad eyes? I agreed to take a look at Luke outside.

Luke's personality sparkled. He smothered me with slobber. Tail flapping, he howled as if belting out a top ten hit. My motorized scooter was no impediment for him although he tried lifting his leg on the rear wheel. Luke handed me his paw, rolled on his back, and kicked his legs in the air. There was no way to resist his canine charm so I adopted him that sweltering July afternoon in 1998.

•

Luke showed potential for pet therapy. I wanted to share his gifts with sick or injured patients, just as Judy and Maxine had uplifted me when my life unexpectedly capsized. My dog breezed through a behavior test and passed a medical examination, allowing us to join the Companion Animal Association of Arizona (CAA), a requirement for therapy work. We were assigned to visit sick, elderly, or injured patients at a rehab center starting in the fall.

My experiences with pet therapy, however, started long before I moved to Arizona. In 1989, I began my shelter career as a volunteer with the MSPCA in Boston. The MSPCA ran a pet therapy program. The animal/human bond had always intrigued me so I enrolled my rescued dog Maxine. I expected her wagging tail and gleaming eyes would bring cheer to dozens of patients. Back then, the guidelines were less stringent. Certification by a national organization wasn't required.

A shelter supervisor met Maxine, determined her to be good with strangers and well behaved. My dog's hardscrabble life on the mean streets of NY didn't turn her surly or nasty. She loved everyone. The MSPCA approved Maxine and assigned us to visit a nursing home in Cambridge then called Neville Manor.

Maxine and I settled into a routine. We visited with seniors, many of whom owned pets before age or illness robbed their independence. Older people shared stories about treasured dogs and cats now entrusted to the care of friends and relatives. For those without resources, the hapless animals ended up in shelters like the MSPCA. Just about everyone had a hard luck story about family who didn't visit, a beloved spouse who passed, or a creeping illness that zapped their spirit. I dreaded getting old or sick. I never imagined that just five years later I'd be using a motorized scooter myself and fearful of the future. Would I too end up in a nursing home?

One senior named Pearl adored Maxine and saved treats for her. At first, I cringed, watching Maxine scarf down the goodies including apple pie, tuna sandwiches, and vanilla wafers. Soon, I came up with a sensible alternative.

"Maxine likes the special treats you give her, Pearl," I said. "But she really needs to stick with dog food. It's better for her."

"Oh," Pearl said, with a pitiful look. "I only wanted to make her happy."

"Of course, you have her interests at heart." I whipped out a few dog biscuits from my pocket. "Give her these. She loves dog cookies. Keep a few for her next visit."

That arrangement worked like a dream and Pearl stopped stuffing my dog with food that wasn't good for her. Maxine of course ate anything in sight but the dog snacks were healthier.

A few residents balked at her visits. One woman screamed every time she saw Maxine and I pass by her room.

"I hate that cat. Don't let that beast into my room," she'd mumble to herself.

I waved and said, "How are you today?" I realized she was either senile or mean spirited. There were so many people to visit. I never bothered to find out what was up with this woman. Maybe I should have?

I moved away from Boston in 1991 but Maxine and I faithfully visited the seniors at Neville Manor for about a year and a half. Saying goodbye was tearful and sad. I'll always remember how my scrappy mutt, once a discard on the mean streets of New York City, brought cheer and joy to seniors in a Boston area nursing home. Maxine left this world in 2001 but I still miss her.

•

On our first week at the Phoenix area nursing home, Luke endeared himself to Kim, the recreation assistant, a gregarious young woman with a Julia Roberts smile. Luke and Kim developed a comical routine that never wavered. At nine every Friday morning, Luke and I arrived and waited in the lobby. As Kim approached, Luke's tail wiggled in circles. He yipped and yowled. I let go of his leash, cracking up as my dog dashed down hall throwing himself into Kim's open arms. My twice abandoned dog was on a roll. So was I.

Patients welcomed us with priceless reactions. Take Maria, the older Latina woman with a brain hobbled by a stroke as an example. Only two words remained in her vocabulary—Maria, Maria. Grinning, she stroked Luke with her good hand and said, "Maria, Maria." I always said hello and asked how she was.

Nodding, she replied, "Maria, Maria." As Luke brushed against her wheelchair, the gleam in eyes showed appreciation. "Maria Maria," she said as I rolled out of her room, always smiling at Luke.

Bald and be-speckled, Will saved treats for Luke, such as bacon strips, hard-boiled eggs, and soggy wheat toast, which my dog gobbled up in seconds. Luke's bad manners tickled Will. The two always interacted with each other good-naturedly. Again, I brought dog biscuits and convinced Will to hand him only these treats on our visits. Two years later, Will had suddenly died. As we bypassed his room, Luke yanked on his leash as if to say, "What about Will?" He missed the old man's affection.

For reasons I never understood, Luke picked Frank as his special friend. Luz, Frank's mother, was stricken with lung and heart disease. In his younger years, Frank drank to excess, was chronically unemployed, and often gambled away his mother's meager earnings as a janitor. Frank finally spruced up his act and visited Luz daily. Every time Luke saw Frank, he bellowed as if he'd seen his best friend. Although Luz was on a ventilator, she smiled at their tender interaction. Several years after I left the rehab center, I drove through a Tempe neighborhood. I noticed Frank outside tending to his lawn. I pulled over to say hello. He invited me inside for an iced tea. There on the couch sat a big fat dog named Budgy. Frank's mother Luz had passed away and I offered my condolences. He took Budgy from a neighbor who no longer wanted the big boy. Frank and his canine companion seemed content. That made my day.

Memory loss hits seniors with a bang. I could relate now that I experienced memory issues. A gray-haired man told me the same story every week about the floppy eared dog he and his late wife found on a lonely country road many years ago. The dog lived with them for a long time and evidently provided them with years of companionship. I never tired of hearing his story although it was the same one, week after week. The man enjoyed Luke's visits and I felt needed. I looked forward to my weekly trips to the home.

Nearly all the patients were elderly except for one, a young man named Mark. He was profoundly brain injured from a drug overdose. Blinking eyes were his only body movements. One blink meant yes;

two was a sign for no. On my first visit, he looked down at my dog as if he wanted to pet him so I guided his hand over Luke's back, moving it back and forth a few times. Unable to smile, a look in his eyes told me he appreciated the gesture. That became our regular routine. One week, we popped into Mark's room and he wasn't there. A nurse said he was in the hospital across the street being treated for an infection. Luke and I visited the hospital before going home. Of course, Mark couldn't speak so we sat in his room and I talked to him like a regular person. Then I heard a voice behind me asking who I was. That was Mark's mother who told me his story. Out on a weekend evening with friends doing drugs a few years ago, Mark apparently overdosed. Frightened by Mark's condition, his friends deserted him. By the time Mark was found, he was almost dead. Paramedics revived him but by then he was severely brain damaged requiring round-the-clock care for the rest of his life. Now pro-active as a result, his mother talked to high school students about the dangers of drug abuse. Mark had a dog that she took care of after the incident. That's why she said her son liked Luke's visits.

Seeing how drugs completely shattered Mark's life reminded me how fortunate I was, never traveling down that road. Yes, I admit to drinking to excess at times and smoking pot but I always shied away from hard drugs. What a blessing that I had such insight to give it all up a long time ago.

Not everyone at the rehab center withered away. Some patients improved and moved into assisted living facilities where pet owner-ship was permitted, sometimes even encouraged, so seniors stayed active and vibrant. Patients asked me for shelter contacts to adopt older cats or dogs for company. I was always glad to help.

Luke not only brightened up patients' lives but he brought relief to over-worked staff too. Nurses, doctors, aides, and therapists benefited from Luke's weekly visits. Everyone loved Luke, especially me. We both had a purpose now.

•

On a blistering summer day in 2001 I stopped at the now closed Bone Appetit dog bakery to buy snacks for my old scraggly hounds. As a shelter volunteer, a steady stream of unwanted dogs found refuge with me. Tasty treats perked them up. At the checkout counter, a newspaper clipping tacked on the wall caught my eye. It was about a doggie beach party. What on earth was this? We're surrounded by the sprawling Sonoran Desert.

"Who had the beach party?" I asked, paying for a bag of pup cakes.

Bakery owner Helen smiled as she explained. "We hosted Gabriel's Angels first fundraiser a few months ago. They're a new therapy dog group that works with abused kids."

Volunteers spent all morning filling up kiddie pools and opening beach umbrellas. Real sand scattered around the parking lot hinted at an ocean feeling. "You should talk to Pam Gaber, the founder." Gaber has since left Gabriel's Angels and remarried but she left behind an amazing organization.

I grabbed Gaber's business card. Over coffee, Gaber sold me on Gabriel's Angels. Luke and I would spread kindness and compassion to heal abused, neglected, and at-risk children. My schedule allowed another weekly visit and Luke was perky enough to handle additional visits.

A group of children gathered around me and Luke shortly after we arrived at the homeless family shelter on our first day. A former motel, the shelter (called LaMesita) was home to about fifty homeless families.

"What's your dog's name?" a seven-year-old boy asked.

"Can I feed him?" a girl with pigtails asked as she giggled when Luke tried to kiss her cheek.

"When does he sleep?" the girl's older brother asked.

"Does Luke watch the Animal Planet?" another boy asked.

That began my seven-year journey with Gabriel's Angels. My life was never the same.

A wheelchair bound boy named Kevin, perhaps nine years old, grabbed my attention. What a place for a disabled kid to end up. Workers said he couldn't talk and I assumed he had cerebral palsy. Kevin grinned when he rolled into the youth center and tried to pet Luke. I guided his hand along Luke's curly fur. Despite staff's assurance that Kevin couldn't talk, I heard words like "Luke" and "the dog." Kevin wasn't there on a subsequent visit so I asked Vaughn, the staff worker, about his absence.

"Where's the boy with CP?"

Vaughn frowned. "Kevin doesn't have CP. His mother's boyfriend beat him up when he was a baby."

Tears swelled in my eyes. "How could he?"

"Evidently the man got enraged when Kevin cried and he kicked him around. Kevin was hurt very badly. He'll be in this chair for life. I'm not sure where he is today."

Memory loss is one of the residual effects from my brain injury but I'll never forget Kevin, the affable, sandy-haired boy in the wheel chair who smiled every time he saw Luke. I regretted that his life was forever marred by violence.

I entered the youth center with Luke one week when Ruth, a girl perhaps twelve years old, flew out of her seat and hugged my dog. A wave of joy swept through me as I watched this girl's reaction.

"A dog. It's really a dog. I'm so happy." Luke returned the affection with generous slobber to the girl's cheek.

"Hi Ruth, I'm Debbie. This is Luke. We visit on Tuesday afternoon."

"I miss having a dog," Ruth said. "I'll love your dog. That's OK, isn't it?"

"Sure, Luke likes everyone."

Through bits and pieces of our interactions, Ruth's damaged psyche became apparent. Her easygoing behavior suddenly turned scary. The other children avoided her, sometimes even mocked her. Even though I'd been a social worker before the accident, I wasn't trained in child psychology but I managed to hold the group together when Ruth acted out. The children didn't understand her emotional anguish. Imprisoned for child abuse, Mom also killed the family dog. Ruth received psychotherapy but the scars penetrated deep into her soul. She often asked if Luke could spend the night. For the three months, Ruth and her father lived at the shelter, we brought a small shred of comfort to a bruised and battered young girl who I hoped was on the road to recovery.

In addition to my work as a pet therapist, I had other volunteer commitments such as answering the phone once a week in former AZ Gov. Janet Napolitano's office. I had once mentioned this to the children. Lacy, about twelve years old, told me how fond she was of the governor. During my tenure with the state, we handed out kid packages upon request. They were facts and figures about Arizona, our government, and the current governor. Upon my next trip to the state house, I asked our supervisor to send a kid package to Lacy, care of the shelter. Apparently, the governor's office had called the shelter to find out the spelling of Lacy's last name. I returned the next week and Lacy was so excited to see me. She said that the governor had called her but she missed the call because she was in school. I didn't have the heart to tell her it wasn't really Janet Napolitano who called but rather someone in her office. Lacy was thrilled to receive the kid pack. And that was my little secret. That small act of kindness went a long way.

Gabriel's Angels handed out stethoscopes to volunteers, compliments of a generous donor. We invited children to listen to the dog's beating heart as a way of spreading compassion.

"He feels pain like you do," I said, watching children line up for a chance to listen. "If someone hits Luke, he hurts. Just like you if you're beaten."

"Hitting a dog is bad," a boy said.

"All violence is bad," I said.

I brought the stethoscope every few weeks. Some children lived at the shelter for the maximum four month stay so I didn't want to lose their attention with the same lesson. I mixed up activities that taught empathy and kindness. The stethoscope, however, was always popular.

•

Teaching compassion and kindness extended beyond animals. A brawl erupted between two pig-tailed third graders while the other children assembled a jigsaw puzzle. I separated the kids and said, "Ladies, please stop fighting. Tell me what this is about."

"She said my mother was a pig," Veronica said, jabbing her finger at Tracy.

"Did not." Tracy lunged at Veronica's throat.

"Did too," Veronica said.

I pressed myself in between the angry girls. "No screaming or hitting. Someone needs to apologize."

Faces gnarled, the two girls wrapped their arms around their chests and huffed.

"Veronica? Tracy? I don't have all day," I said.

There was nothing but silence so I picked up Luke's leash and headed toward the door.

"Where're you going?" wide-eyed Veronica asked. "Is Luke leaving?"

"Luke doesn't like it when you children fuss and fight."

I sighed with relief as Veronica and Tracy quickly made up. I wasn't sure I could defuse the tension but it seems as if I did.

•

A brother and sister from Michigan adored Luke. They missed their dog, Brownie, left behind when the family unit crumbled. Dad failed to keep up child support payments after a bitter divorce. Mom lost her factory job and foreclosure took away their home. The dog went to a neighbor and the family hoped for a new life in Phoenix. Mom, however, couldn't land a job and without Dad's child support, they ended up in the shelter.

One afternoon we discussed grooming dogs and cats and the kids told me a story.

"Mommy was driving home from Auntie's house," Shawn said. "She saw a man beat his dog."

Mom pulled over and asked the man to stop hitting the dog. He did.

"Mommy told him she would take the dog until he could treat him better," Shawn said. "That's how we got Brownie."

Not only did this courageous woman save a dog from brutality but she taught her children a vital lesson about respect and kindness. They learned that it was OK for an adult to intervene when a helpless animal was threatened.

"You're too young to stop animal abuse on your own," I said, "but ask a responsible adult you know or an agency to help." Empowering children was important. Pet therapy empowered me to feel wanted and valued.

•

Children formed strong bonds with Luke and saw him as an ally. Over the years they groomed him, read stories with his paw cradled in their laps, and confided in him as if he was a mentor. They always remembered Luke's name but called me the dog lady. That tickled me. Although some children had been maltreated or had lived in foster care, they often came up with clever ways to help beat up and cast aside animals. Take the helpless kitten found clawing her way out of a bush tucked behind the shelter. Jessie, a fifth grader, greeted me at the door with "big news." Cool sunny weather permitted supervised outside play. Desperate meows caught Jessie's attention. She followed the squeaky voice until she found a kitten stuck inside a leafy bush. Remembering what I said about animals in need, Jessie called to the supervisor, a young woman named Margie.

"You said to get an adult for an animal in need," Jessie said, sitting up proudly.

"You remembered," I said.

"Margie picked the kitten from the bushes and brought her inside. We all helped clean her up." Animal lover Margie had room for one more animal in her multi-pet household. The children were so proud of themselves.

•

Due to the vagaries of shelter life, homeless children often lagged in school. Large families may be cramped into one or two small rooms, depriving children of quiet time for studies. With Luke as the focus, I often brought flash cards to bolster their learning. No sooner had I whipped out the math cards when Stevie, a twelve-year-old, started to cry. Surely, it couldn't be the math so I asked, "What's wrong?"

In between sniffles, Stevie said, "My brother and I got beat up on the school bus today."

Down with the flash cards; math would wait. "What happened?"

A group of poorly-behaved girls picked on the brothers on because they lived at a homeless shelter. Stevie and his freckle-face brother John were both shy, slightly built boys. So, when the female warriors pounced on them, the boys didn't fight back. None of the other students intervened either. The bus driver, according to the boys, said nothing.

Vaughn called the school principal to discuss the pressing matter. I led a discussion among the children present about bullying. Why it happened? How it can be prevented? What to do if you are a victim?

On my way out, Luke sidled up next to puffy-eyed Stevie. He rested his paw in the boy's lap. I hugged him and said I was sorry. I didn't know what else to do.

•

Every Christmas, a friend volunteered with an organization that collected toys for children in need. Another friend bought toys for the children on her own. I wrapped each child's gift in holiday paper and a bow. Their excitement was priceless as they ripped open the presents and treated them as if they were gold. As a bonus, I borrowed Christmas music CDs from the library. We sang along to tunes such as "Jingle Bells," "Silent Night," and "Hark the Herald Angels Sing." Luke added his own canine crooning by howling at various parts of the songs. That made the children crack up. Christmas at a homeless shelter instead of your own home was a sobering experience. Shelter staff and volunteers pitched in to make their holiday as warm and comforting as possible.

At times, I felt so inadequate, helpless even. So many troubled children passed through with emotional anguish that stretched beyond my position as a pet therapist. Even my training as a social worker didn't always give me an advantage and I relied on Luke to soothe their wounded souls. But there were times even my dog couldn't help.

A single mother, Linda, and her eight children arrived after an eviction. Rage and bitterness swirled around Linda nearly every time she opened her mouth. She didn't speak; she bellowed. The oldest, Angela who was about twelve, served as a surrogate parent to her large brood. Nearly all her children acted out by fighting with others, refusing to obey rules. Some of them related to Luke but whenever I was around, I spent most of my time breaking up spats. Talks about non-violence and harmony sailed over their heads. The staff worker shared a few tidbits about Linda. At twelve, she gave birth to Angela. Since then, she'd been pregnant nearly every other year. Few, if any, of the children's fathers were in their lives. She had trouble holding a job. In fact, the day we spoke, the shelter delivered another blow. In ten days, Linda had to be out for failure to comply with the rules. Despite the odds against finding a place for her large brood, Linda pulled off a miracle. I never saw the family again. I didn't enjoy a close family relationship growing up but at least I never experienced rape or incest. I always hoped that Linda and her children found healing.

•

On December 26, 2004, tragedy struck half way around the world. A giant tsunami nearly swallowed up Asian countries like Thailand, Sri Lanka, and Indonesia. Thousands of people died while the monster storm left millions without homes. Wrecked commerce left millions without jobs. The news jolted me. I could hardly believe the terrible images of death and destruction.

Moved by the frightful situation I shared my thoughts with the children. Despite being homeless, their hearts were full of empathy for the lives shattered by the tsunami. With little help from me, they wrote letters to ambassadors of the most severely impacted countries. I added cover letters explaining who we were and mailed them to the United Nations. A few weeks later, my phone rang. I almost didn't answer. The ambassador's office from Sri Lanka called to thank me for the kind and thoughtful note the children sent. As soon as the country recovered from the massive devastation, she would read our letters to schools across the country. I felt so honored. I returned the next week with the good news. A few children who signed the letters had moved. Too bad they weren't around to hear the personal message from Sri Lanka. I'm sorry I didn't keep copies of the letters. I just have the memories.

•

I brought Beanie Baby dolls to play a pretend game of compassion to animals. Instead, a group of children played violent games with the stuffed animals, beating them, and slamming them against the table. Their sudden outbursts startled me. Maybe these children had experienced violence at home.

"Stop that, please," I said. "I brought these dolls so you kids could have something fuzzy to cuddle and learn about compassion. Please don't act out games that hurt."

A few children continued to act mean spirited despite my pleas to behave gently. Finally, I said, "That's it. Give them back. All of them. I come here to spread kindness and compassion."

No one said a word as I collected the dolls. On my way out, children not involved in violent games asked me if they could have the dolls back. I said yes but only if they played with them nicely.

•

The children never asked me for anything, except once. A boy named Marshall, perhaps twelve years old, asked if he could live with me. After the initial surprise, I asked him why. First, he loved dogs and wanted so much to have a dog of his own. But the real reason was deeper, more than just a love of dogs. Marshall was ashamed of his single mother. His five siblings all had different fathers. At that time, his mother had another boyfriend. She wasn't pregnant but Marshall figured she would have another baby with the new boyfriend, who he didn't like. Sometimes, the children at school poked fun of him because of his family situation. He didn't know how to defend himself or his mother. Caught off guard, I told Marshall I was sorry about his troubles but I couldn't raise him. I asked about living arrangements with his father or other family members. He didn't know his father so that wasn't possible. I then suggested talking to the school counselor. Maybe she could at least help with the classmate's bad behavior. My heart broke for Marshall. To this day, I think about him sometimes and hope that his life worked out OK.

•

Every summer the shelter asked me to extend my weekly visits. I always said yes. I looked for interesting and educational opportunities. I prodded the owner of a local yoga parlor to offer free yoga lessons for the kids. I arranged a visit to Whole Foods, a natural grocery store. A worker guided us through the huge facility, explaining natural foods and healthy living. At the end of our visit each child received a gift bag filled with wholesome snacks. We toured a ranch for abused and unwanted horses. The kids related to horses that didn't have homes. I invited speakers from the Sierra Club to talk about our natural environment and how they could be kinder to Mother Nature. A woman who raised guide dogs for the blind showed us how the dogs were trained. A sheriff's deputy from Maricopa County talked about animal abuse. And the Arizona Puppet Theater put on a fabulous, entertaining performance every year that made the kids laugh, smile and giggle.

At the end of 2008, Luke and I retired as a therapy team. Age had crept up on Luke. My dog had to be at least twelve years old, although he could have been older. I just didn't know. His spirits were as sunny as ever but he had slowed down, showing more interest in curling up for a good snooze than interacting with the kids.

During sessions kids would ask me, "Why does Luke sleep so much?" One boy laughed at Luke's snoring.

Seven years as a pet therapist changed my life. Employers rejected my applications for part-time jobs but I felt valued for my pet therapy work. I experienced the hardships of old age as well as homelessness. I experienced the rupture of family ties. I sensed the children's pain as they talked of loss. Homelessness involves leaving behind good friends, familiar neighborhoods, beloved pets, and comfortable schools. Living in shelters and nursing homes among strangers can be scary. Talk of family violence unsettled me. I taught children negotiating skills to get along in the world without whacking someone. I hope they listened. Luke cuddled with them. He kissed a few cheeks. He rested his paw on kids and elders who sat alone. We cared, we loved, and we extended ourselves to make a difference to children who needed us. I also felt the sadness in seniors confined to a congregate care facility. Losing their independence as well as their homes was a heavy burden. Some lost pets too. I hope their world is better because we were there.

Luke died from massive seizures in January, 2010. I'll always miss the dog nobody wanted. He was truly the best.

Chapter Eleven

John Kerry's 2004 Presidential Campaign

In 2004, the USA was heavily immersed in, what I considered, illegal, immoral, and unethical wars in both Afghanistan and Iraq. We only now have a small presence in Iraq. Troops left Afghanistan in 2021. Then President George W. Bush did not represent my values or feelings as an American. His bid for re-election worried me so I volunteered for the John Kerry campaign, his Democratic opponent. That was my first exposure with a political campaign. From August right up until the November Election Day, I was a regular volunteer in John Kerry's East Valley campaign office. Staff and volunteers welcomed me and made me feel valuable I was thrilled to be part of a team. Twice weekly, I made telephone calls asking Democratic voters if they were registered. I provided information on how to register if they were not. I don't recall if there was online registration back then. A subsequent round of calls involved asking voters if they received their mail-in ballots. We encouraged those interested to sign up for early voting. Follow-up calls were made to ask if voters filled out their ballots and if they had in fact actually mailed them. We asked if voters needed rides to the polls on election day. We were instructed to be polite and courteous, even if a voter said they planned to vote for Bush.

"Thank you for your time," I said to my first Bush supporter.

"Don't you want to know why I'm voting for Bush?" the voter asked.

"Sure, go ahead."

"I don't care how many innocent people or American soldiers get killed overseas. Bush is against abortion. So am I. That's why he gets my vote."

Wow, I was speechless but managed to cough up a few words and said, "Have a nice day."

Voter reaction to abortion ran from support to lack of concern to extreme. I had just talked to an extremist, perhaps someone who supported bombing of abortion clinics or violence against doctors who performed abortions. I support a woman's right to choose and hope we can always keep abortion safe and legal in this country in spite of a setback from the Supreme Court.

I asked another voter about registering early. She simply said, "We don't vote."

I wondered who *we* were so I asked.

"Jehovah's Witnesses don't vote."

"Oh," I said. "Thanks for your time."

I never knew that before. Every US citizen should vote but that's my personal opinion.

At one point, our record keeping volunteers were late inputting data from our calls. A woman I reached on the phone huffed and puffed. "If I get another call from the Kerry campaign, I swear I'm voting for Bush. Stop calling me."

I asked the computer volunteers to please update their records so we didn't place repeat calls.

Volunteers like me did everything possible to assure that Democrats or independents voted for John Kerry. As each week passed, more volunteers flocked to our tiny office and offered their help. Some dropped in to give moral support or to pick up a Kerry for president lawn sign or bumper sticker. There were reports of vandalism with Kerry signs either being stolen or defaced. Toward the end of the campaign, we asked for a small contribution to replace the many signs we handed out.

A group of German tourists once popped in to chat. They asked how could anyone vote for Bush. In unison, all the volunteers shrugged and said we didn't know. Those tourists left with Kerry bumper stickers. During my short time on the Kerry campaign trail, I came to know good, decent people who wanted the best for our country. I was proud to work among so many dedicated and caring Americans of all races, ages, and nationalities. On election night, all the Democrats gathered at a hotel in downtown Phoenix to watch the returns. By 11:00 p.m. it was clear the numbers weren't going our way. All of us were saddened and blue. I didn't know whether to scream or cry. As we know, Bush went on to serve a second term. Campaign volunteers gathered the next night for a pizza party at a local restaurant to say goodbye. Now and then I run into someone from the Kerry campaign. It's always a pleasure to see a long-lost colleague who shares my values and spirit. The excitement of the campaign, however, spurred my interest in politics.

In addition to the Kerry campaign, I also volunteered on several other Democratic campaigns, such as Jim Pederson's attempt to unseat Republican Jon Kyl in 2006. Although the entire team gave it a valiant effort, Kyl went on to serve another term before retiring in 2012. The year 2006 was a busy one for me politically. I also volunteered for Governor Janet Napolitano who sought a second term that she won. Similar to the Kerry campaign, we worked from voter registration lists. We asked Democrats if they were registered to vote. Negative replies were given information on how to register. Follow-up calls were made. Then we asked about voting by mail and gave out information on how to do so. We also made follow-up calls. As the election neared, we called voters to ask if they filled out their ballots. The aim of course was to ensure a Democratic victory.

Undoubtedly GOP volunteers did the same for our rivals. From my limited experience working on political campaigns, I discovered an incredible energy among volunteers who were eager for change. At the time in 2006, the USA was in the midst of bitter, protracted Middle East wars in Iraq and Afghanistan where Americans as well as Iraqis and Afghani's suffered heavy losses. Americans were finally turning against the wars and wanted change but apparently not enough because the GOP still retained sizable control of Congress. I served among proud, energetic, and capable Arizona residents who just wanted to live in peace.

We're still involved in Middle East wars and the world is not at peace. The campaign experience uplifted me and gave me hope that plenty of people in our community cared about our world enough to spend countless hours of their own time to make it a better world. Thank you, everyone, for the joys and tears we experienced during those many evenings working the phones to get people up and out to vote. I'll never forget those days. Not ever.

Chapter Twelve
Governor Janet Napolitano's Office of Constituent Services

Volunteering for the Kerry campaign was thrilling. After it ended, the energy lived on and I wondered what to do. I searched around and called Governor Janet Napolitano's office to see if they had a volunteer program. Sure enough, they did and I asked about joining it. The manager at the time, the late Melodee Jackson, invited me to her office for an introductory meeting. By the end of our talk, I agreed to volunteer every Monday morning. The work mostly involved answering the phone, sorting through mail for filing, and other projects as needed.

"Governor Napolitano's office, may I help you?" I said, greeting our first caller to Janet Napolitano's office.

"A spirit named Misty invaded my body. I need $600 to remove the spirit," the woman said as if asking a friend for a handout. "The guide wants the money up front and no one will lend it to me. Not my mother, not my sister, no one. Can I get it from the governor?"

No, I said. Psychological counseling was more prudent than a costly medium. She balked at the idea. Furious that the state of Arizona wouldn't hand over $600 for spirit removal, the caller slammed down the phone. Was this a sign of things to come?

That started a typical morning as a volunteer in Janet Napolitano's office of constituent services. Once weekly, I answered calls from residents, nearly all from Arizona although calls sometimes filtered in from California, Michigan, and other states.

During my second week in November 2004, a caller asked for Janet. I didn't recall meeting anyone named Janet. Quickly, I sorted through the people I'd met. There was Carolyn, Melodee, Ezra, Betty Sue, but I couldn't remember anyone named Janet. So I asked, "Janet who?"

The caller shot back, "The governor, you idiot."

The caller wanted legal advice from Janet Napolitano who had served as state attorney general from 1998–2002. Prior to that, she served as a US Attorney and was in private practice. I said the governor didn't give legal advice on the phone. The small business owner hadn't paid rent and faced eviction proceedings.

"I suggest you contact a lawyer. The state can't help you, I'm sorry," I said.

The caller grumbled a few words then hung up. In December, volunteers shared a holiday lunch with the governor and I told that story. The governor laughed.

Sometimes it took mere seconds to determine a call was unrelated to Arizona. A woman wanted the governor to "use her influence" to move up her passport request. She made vacation plans not long after the Bush administration imposed stringent requirements on foreign travel. Americans now needed passports to visit both Canada and Mexico. Deluged with passport and visa requests, the State Department warned citizens to apply months in advance because of processing backlogs. Some travelers shrugged off warnings and booked last minute travel plans anyway. Airline tickets to foreign countries without passports and/or visas were useless. Pressure tactics on our office didn't work. Despite glowing comments such as "the governor can do anything" or "I really like Janet," we told callers the governor had no influence over the State Department. We suggested calling their Congressional delegation.

Another caller wanted the governor for an urgent matter.

"The governor doesn't take calls from the public. That's the purpose of the office of constituent services. I'll try to help you," I said.

"Tell her that God blesses her. He won't bless you though because you won't let me talk to her."

I didn't take it personally as I chuckled to myself.

A man from out of state claims the state of Arizona blocked his ability to work. "Why?" I asked. The irate caller received a traffic ticket in Arizona a few years ago.

"I paid it, of course," he said. "You people didn't get your records straight. When I tried to renew my license, which I need to drive, they said I owe the ticket. This is an outrage. I have a family to feed. What're you going to do?"

"Did you call the Department of Motor Vehicles?"

"The phone lines are constantly busy."

As a rule, I referred callers to the appropriate department for resolution. As an alternative, they could write the governor for further investigation. This time, however, I wilted and offered to look into his problem.

"What county were you ticketed?" I asked.

"Solano."

"Sir, there is no Solano County in Arizona."

"It says right here, Solano County."

I asked him to read the ticket to me. I moved to Arizona in 1997 so I wasn't entirely familiar with the state's geography but I knew that Solano County didn't exist.

"Maybe it's a town called Solano," he said.

"That's a big help. Let me do some checking and I'll call you back."

The man omitted a few salient points. He had paid the ticket late last Friday afternoon, not years ago. The county clerk, who worked alone in a rural part of Arizona, didn't have time to process his credit card payment until sometime later on Monday or Tuesday. Because I called on behalf of the governor's office she offered to rush through his paperwork.

"Take your time," I said. "This guy lied. Process the payment at your regular schedule. I'll call him back and tell him it'll be done today or tomorrow."

When I confronted Mr. Late Payment, he sounded miffed. I reminded him that Arizona wasn't responsible for his inability to renew his driver's license—he was. I vowed I wouldn't make any more calls for constituents as many only told us bits and pieces of the truth. But I always filled out an intake form on everyone who called including the people who got on my nerves.

I relented one more time and called a city agency for a constituent who was a snowbird. Snowbirds are senior citizens who live in Arizona during the winter but leave when the temperature rises to the triple digits. Some live in Canada. The caller, now in Utah, said the city of Superior was crushing his civil rights. How unfair, he claimed. The city removed his mobile home from a private park without consent and his rights were violated. The city, he said, wasn't returning his calls. I asked him for contact info. I called and reached a manager right away. The park issued numerous safety violations to the snowbird for his mobile home, which was in shambles. Mr. Snowbird ignored them all. The city of Superior mailed him a notice saying his mobile home would be towed off the property unless he made the required repairs. The letter was sent return receipt requested. The city had the receipt proving Mr. Snowbird had received it. When confronted, he admitted that he was in violation but said he didn't think it should apply to him. I said he'd have to take up matters with the city. The state of Arizona was no longer involved.

A woman called to say the state of Arizona raped her. A bit extreme but I listened as I always did. Middle-aged and maybe lonely, she opened a joint bank account with a new boyfriend she met online. The boyfriend neglected to reveal he owed a bundle in child support arrears. The state finds the account and seizes the money, which is perfectly legal. The woman is irate yet she's still with the boyfriend. She wants the governor to return her money. I told her to take up the matter with the Department of Economic Security, Child Support Division, or to hire a lawyer. The governor's office could not intervene in a private matter like this.

I picked up the phone and a caller said, "Janet. Is that you?" We had a lot of those. Callers sometimes actually thought I was Janet Napolitano and that she answered her own phone. Momentarily, I felt upbeat being mistaken for the governor.

A local woman from NJ called about slow services in Arizona. She wanted to speak to the governor. She didn't explain what particular services were slow. When I said a personal conversation with the governor wasn't possible, the caller became upset. She said she was moving back to NJ to be with her own kind.

Hard luck cases often found their way to our office. Sometimes we could help; sometimes we could not. A recently unemployed woman called with a pickle of a story. The Department of Economic Security denied her unemployment application because of identity theft. To qualify, the caller had to file a police report then request an administrative hearing. She would probably qualify for benefits but the process might string along months. In such cases, there was nothing we could do. What a double whammy—she loses her job then runs up against a thief who stole her identity. To exacerbate matters, she could not collect unemployment insurance either until the case was resolved.

Now and then the calls were absurd. "What's the name of the governor's psychic?"

"Excuse me?" I said.

"The governor's psychic. What's her name?"

"The state of Arizona doesn't employ a psychic." Such calls needed my patience and lots of it.

"That's not what I heard. It's a waste of taxes."

"Where did you get that information?"

The caller hung up. I wanted to know who spread that rumor so we could squash it. A lot of weird calls came in. Some amused me while others were just stupid.

A woman called in a panic. Her husband, a heart transplant recipient, had been receiving AHCCCS, Arizona's version of Medicaid. His application for Social Security Disability was recently approved thus edging his income over AHCCCS strict limits. The state just paid for his heart transplant but would no longer cover lifesaving rejection medication because Social Security. Social Security Disability recipients don't receive Medicare for another two years. Another volunteer worked the phones for several hours that morning, trying to find a solution. The Arizona Heart Hospital that performed the surgery kept an emergency pharmaceutical supply. After we came up empty, the hospital offered to supply the rejection drugs unless another arrangement could be made. No matter how we tried to calm this woman, she was sure her beloved husband would die.

The governor sometimes traveled to Mexico to promote trade with Arizona. Trade created jobs at home and in Mexico, increasing tax revenue for both sides. Not everyone saw it as a boost to the economy. A woman with a chip on her shoulder the size of a Buick said promoting trade with Mexico violated the US Constitution. As she rattled off parts of the Constitution, I politely interrupted her and said, "My shorthand skills are limited. You're free to write to the governor either through email or snail mail to express your views." She shrugged me off and reminded me that promoting trade with Mexico was illegal and that Janet Napolitano should not make any more state sponsored trips to "that" country.

Parents and family members often asked Gov. Napolitano to personally defray the cost of their children's tuition, medical expenses, dance lessons, or summer camp. One woman owed back taxes and wanted the governor to kick in toward her unpaid balance. Others represented charities and wanted the governor to contribute. Undoubtedly, the governor had her own charities but that was her business.

Self-important people wanted to convey ideas directly to the governor. I offered a sound alternative, such as contacting the head of a particular department but to some, that wasn't good enough. They insisted on talking directly to Janet Napolitano. If I couldn't produce a direct line or personal email they threatened to report me for insubordination. Some did just that and I once got chewed out for being nasty. I defended the state of Arizona and I defended Janet Napolitano but I was never rude to anyone.

A volunteer returned a constituent's call by leaving a message on his machine. He called back and insisted it was Janet Napolitano who had called. I assured him it was not.

"Sir, it was someone from our office," I said. "We call everyone back in a timely fashion."

"No, the governor called me. I want to speak to her."

"She doesn't return these calls. That's what we do."

"I'll just wait for her call." I said to myself, he'll be waiting for one heck of a long time.

One woman called for the governor's personal intervention in her husband's criminal case. Recently sentenced to a long term for his third drunk driving conviction, the man would serve a long time. Arizona imposes stiff penalties for driving under the influence. The single mother of two feared crushing poverty without his income. "What am I going to do? I can't make it alone."

"I'm very sorry," I said. "The governor can't undo his sentence. That would be illegal. I can refer you for public assistance. That's about all I can offer."

I heard sniffling. "Please don't do this," she pleaded. "I need him."

There was a strong chance she would drift into poverty, maybe even become homeless, but the state couldn't intervene. Some situations left me feeling like a heel.

Illegal immigration from our southern border framed Gov. Janet Napolitano's tenure and thrust her into the national spotlight. Local and national television invited her to discuss immigration and how Arizona confronted it. In Washington, DC, she pressed former President George W. Bush for National Guard troops and an increase in Border Patrol agents. In 2007, she signed a controversial state law that would sever the license of a business that knowingly hired undocumented workers. Intense pressure built from citizens, the legislature, local officials, and the business community to deal with illegal immigration. No matter what the governor did or didn't do, someone was always unhappy. Take the man who called to complain about the governor's state of the state address. He said it didn't include immigration.

"Sir, it's only 10:00 a.m. The governor hasn't given the speech yet," I said.

"Oh," he said, in a thick foreign accent.

"Well, she better include it."

"Bet she will."

Undocumented citizens from Mexico in search of jobs and a way to escape grinding poverty streamed across the porous US–Mexican border. For years, immigrants entered the US for low-wage jobs as laborers, construction workers, and in agriculture. Most raised families and blended into the community. Their children attended school and ate at McDonald's. When gang violence involving Latinos tore apart neighborhoods and the US economy soured, demand for immigration reform increased. For hardliners that only meant deportation. Our office took calls demanding the governor seal the border with troops. Others wanted an electrical fence. One man called and said he had a simple solution. "Shoot everyone who crosses the border and ask questions later." A woman called and demanded to know why the National Guard couldn't secure the boarder by stand "shoulder to shoulder" along the entire Arizona–Mexico border. I always said I'd pass along your comments to the governor but once in a while that wasn't good enough. They wanted immediate action to quell their anger.

"What's *she* doing to do about it? I want those illegals out and I want them out now."

Even children got into the act. A grammar school child wrote a letter where he suggested digging a moat between the US and Mexico and filling it with snakes, scorpions, and other "creepy things." Some people unabashedly suggested emptying animal shelters of unwanted pit bulls and using them to attack undocumented immigrants as they crossed. The venom in people's voices scared me. I hoped the US never followed the genocide in Rwanda.

Some calls amused me. A woman with a thick Slavic accent wanted a phone number in the Phoenix city government. I didn't like enabling people but I looked anyway.

"Do you have a phone book at home?" I asked.

"No, only one from Bucharest," she said.

I laughed to myself. "May I suggest you call Qwest and ask for a phone book. They're free." Qwest (now Century Link) was the telephone company that served the Phoenix area at the time.

Soldiers returning from Iraq and Afghanistan often called the office seeking help obtaining services from the Veteran's Administration. The VA is a Federal agency so we generally referred them to then Senator Kyl or Senator McCain or their House Representative. A soldier's wife called and wanted help with a problem. After listening to her, the wife was trying to use her husband's military service to garner my sympathy. The couple owned a house in Florida that was part of a homeowner's association. Part of the HOA agreement called for regular maintenance which they evidently ignored. So the HOA slapped them with fines, which had increased. The wife wanted the governor to intervene with the Florida HOA to have the fines tossed out. I said we could not do that. Maintaining a home was their responsibility.

Another soldier, an Arizona citizen, returning from Iraq called to speak with the governor personally. I went through my usual routine and asked him how we could help him. He racked up several speeding and parking tickets before heading out to Iraq. He had ignored them. In his absence, not surprisingly the fines added up. He wanted the governor to step in and have the tickets tossed out. I said we cannot do that. He would have to deal with the city of Scottsdale himself.

A man asked me if I'd heard about the Rumsfeld report. "Excuse me?" I said, totally caught off guard. Donald Rumsfeld was the secretary of defense at the time.

The Rumsfeld report, he said. "Have you read it?"

He supposedly obtained a copy of a confidential arms report that was vital to national security interests. "I'm prepared to sell missiles to the state of Arizona."

"Missiles!" I exclaimed. I could hardly believe this. Only the Armed Forces buy missiles, I said. Arizona isn't in the market for weaponry, no matter how cheaply you can sell them. He hung up and I immediately went into Melodee Jackson's office, the department director. I told her that if the governor approved, I could get a sweet deal on missiles. We both laughed.

A man calling himself an apostle wanted to speak to the governor. He offered a cure for one of the many droughts that plagued Arizona.

"Speaking to Gov. Napolitano personally isn't possible but you can leave a message," I said.

"Then the drought will continue and it's your fault." I didn't lose sleep that night.

On a relatively peaceful day with mostly routine call, an irate man calls and wants to talk to the governor. No bank will approve a loan on a condemned house. He wants the state to lend him the money.

"The state doesn't lend money," I said.

"It's a great investment I'll have to pass up," he said. "I really need the governor. She'd agree this is a good deal."

The conversation ended with me passing along his comments about the fabulous deal that slipped through his fingers because Arizona wouldn't lend him money.

The rich and famous sought help from Governor Napolitano too. A relative of a high-ranking official in the Bush administration asked me if I recognized her name. I did. She asked to speak with the governor. I handed her my usual response and I offered to help.

"It's personal. I'd like to talk to her." Convicted of a DUI, she wanted the governor to intervene. I asked if she had a lawyer. She didn't like the deal he arranged and thought the governor might smooth something more to her liking. I told Melodee, the office director. The governor's chief of staff called her attorney, warning him never to call again asking for special favors.

The governor spoke at dozens of public events and talked to hundreds of Arizona residents across the state. She often gave out our telephone number in the event she couldn't answer a question. Friendly and amiable, that's what made her popular. A woman called one day and said she'd met the governor at some public event. She wanted to talk to her. The governor probably met thousands of Arizona citizens since she's been in office. She can't possibly remember them all. The caller spoke as if they were best friends since high school. I said I'd relay a message. I was convinced that if they were such good friends, she'd have the governor's private number, which we had no access to. The caller didn't sound satisfied but that was the best I could do.

The governor's office received many letters from children. Melodee said the governor enjoyed reading their letters. Once in a while, the governor picked out letters and called the children personally. That must've really thrilled the children when they heard, "The governor is calling."

Each child who wrote received a Kid's Pack containing information about the governor, state history, Arizona landmarks, and how to remain safe.

Another rumor spread among Christian churches that the state planned to give preferential treatment to Muslim students in public schools. Our office was deluged with letters angrily demanding that no such action be taken. None of this of course was true. We had no idea where the rumor started either.

Someone called from California and didn't get the response they wanted. She said, "I'm calling Gov. Arnold Schwarzenegger from California. He'll help me."

Sometimes, we sorted through the governor's mail. Prisoners sent dozens of letters asking for a way out of jail. Nearly all proclaimed innocence. A few said they'd join the army and serve in Iraq if the governor released them. Others swore they found religion and if released, they'd serve God and never again get in trouble.

Out of all the letters a handful of prisoners were perhaps wrongly convicted. They had to pursue their cases through the criminal justice system, not the governor's office. Some letters made me laugh while others I felt like shredding. A few were clever, such as an inmate serving a life sentence in California on a "three strikes, you're out" offense. If the native Arizonan had committed his crimes in our state and not California, he'd be eligible for parole in a few years, not serving life. He asked Gov. Napolitano for a transfer to an Arizona prison so he could be released in the near future. I fell out laughing. There was no way that would happen. Too bad he wasted his talent and would spend his life in jail.

The 2008 presidential election was a tumultuous time. Gov. Napolitano campaigned for Obama, much to the disappointment of Clinton supporters. Some called and said that Janet Napolitano owed her political career to Bill Clinton who appointed her as US Attorney in 1993. They felt she was obligated to support Hillary. Some female callers insisted they'd never vote for the governor if she ran for national office. Other callers wanted to know how much of the state's money the governor spent stumping around for Obama. I told them all the same thing.

"The Obama campaign pays her expenses," I said. "No state tax dollars are used."

After Obama won the election, a woman called and was just furious. She could hardly speak. "How do I sell my citizenship? I don't want to be an American anymore." I told her to call the State Department.

Each Christmas, children from Valley schools were invited to sing songs in front of the Capitol tree. Family and friends sat in chairs. The children added a festive touch to the often-testy mood at the Capitol. Sometimes the governor's office had children from across the state make ornaments for the tree.

On the day of the tree lighting ceremony, a large crowd gathered, including school children, their families, state employees, and visitors. The media surrounded the tree and waited for the governor to make her grand entrance. She lit the tree to a hearty round of applause. Then, she made a short speech and wished everyone a happy holiday.

In mid-September 2007, I left that Monday as usual around noon. I said goodbye to Melodee, who was finishing lunch. Before she headed out for her after meal smoke, I said, "See you next week."

"We'll be here," was her typical response.

The next Monday she wasn't there. During a casual dinner with her sister, she collapsed and never regained consciousness. She died September 21. At her funeral, which was attended by hundreds, I cried as the governor talked about their special friendship. Melodee Jackson and Janet Napolitano had formed a friendship around twenty years earlier when Melodee was head of the fledgling Arizona Democratic Party and Janet Napolitano, an attorney in private practice, served as their legal counsel. Melodee was a wonderful, thoughtful human being who served the state well for many years. The office was much duller after she passed. I missed her wisdom, her caring, and her concern for Arizona and all the people who lived here.

Janet Napolitano resigned in January 2009 to become Secretary of Homeland Security in the Obama administration. Serving Arizona for all those years was a rewarding experience. I dressed up for my shift and felt as if I made a difference. I enjoyed working with my colleagues. Every now and then, I saw the governor in the parking lot. She always waved to me. A day at the office was always a pleasure as well as a challenge. Calls were mostly ordinary but some tested our resolve. I referred people to various government agencies. I listened to them complain. Once in a while, I hung up on rude, obnoxious, and offensive callers. But the experience uplifted me in ways I didn't expect. I met lots of interesting, fun, and sometimes crotchety people. Public service made me proud to call Arizona home.

Chapter Thirteen

The Department of Economic Security, Child Support Division

For about nine months to a year after I left the governor's office, I volunteered once a week in the Child Support Division of the Arizona Department of Economic Security, also known as DES.

That huge state bureaucracy deals with welfare, healthcare, food stamps, child protective services, and child support among other human services. Mostly I sorted through legal papers then placed them inside individual's files. Documents about place of employment, bank accounts, etc. were retained because child support cases often ended up in court. Such routine tasks were boring but I met interesting people. Plus, volunteering gave me a reason to get out of bed, wear decent clothes, and leave the house. Volunteer work boosted my self-esteem. Letter writers to the *Arizona Republic*, our daily newspaper, often chastised state employees as lazy, shiftless, and unworthy of merit increases. That's not what I saw during my time at DES or the governor's office. Employees dedicated themselves to tracking down deadbeat dads and in some cases moms who didn't pay child support. There was a system in place to obtain the employers, bank accounts (if any), and addresses of deadbeat parents, most of whom were men. Now and then, the absent parent was a woman and DES pursued her with the same vigor.

Each worker in the process performed the needed steps to collect the arrears and they were tireless in their efforts. Seizing large amounts of past due child support from deadbeat parents who won the lottery or hit it big from a lawsuit was seen as a sense of pride from state workers. But most cases were not as thrilling and instead were routine. Sometimes the state was successful in collecting from uncooperative parents, usually through wage attachments. Other times they arranged a court-ordered repayment plan. Some mothers eagerly cooperated with DES by providing the father's place of employment, Social Security number, address, phone, etc., making the state's job easier. Other mothers, however, were reticent. They claimed to have no information about the father's whereabouts even though in some cases DES discovered they were living together. And then there was the case of fathers who fell behind in child support payments because of illness, loss, or employment or re-marriage. The state was adamant and accepted no excuses especially in the case of a new marriage. That wasn't their problem if dad remarried and had additional children. He was still responsible to repay child support or arrearages. He could, of course, petition the court to lower his support commitments but usually judges were unsympathetic. If a father lost his job or was imprisoned, the state had little option. As the old adage goes, you cannot get blood from a stone. Without an income, there is no wage to attach. In those situations, the arrears built up. Mothers sometimes could squeeze by without the support. Sometimes they could not. Life was unfair sometimes.

The child support division only chased down fathers who owed child support if a mother received Aid to Families with Dependent Children (AFDC) benefits. The state wanted its money back and it was the absent parent's responsibility to payback the taxpayers of Arizona. The child support division didn't handle private matters concerning child support between two feuding parents. In that case, an outside attorney had to become involved.

In addition to filing, my volunteer work also introduced me to the soap opera of people's personal lives. One man had fathered ten children, including one in Arizona. Nine states pursued him for failure to pay child support. Arizona wanted him, but the state was too late. Another state beat them to him. No matter how much money a person owes, courts only allow one wage attachment at a time. Everyone else has to wait in line. Theoretically, a deadbeat can have attachments lined up against him until retirement age. It seemed doubtful Arizona would ever collect the money this man owed.

Some men, angered over the break-up of a failed marriage or relationship, retaliate on their ex-wives or girlfriends by moving from job to job or working off the books so that the courts never catch up with them to serve child support orders. Fathers who failed to pay child support often pushed women into poverty. Children are hurt through no fault of their own. From the files I sorted through, some dads failed to pay because they were imprisoned. Others fled the country. Once in a while, a man denied paternity altogether. In that case, the state gave the accused a chance to prove or disprove paternity through a simple blood test. If he could not keep the appointment, he had better call to cancel with a good reason. Failure to show up was automatically considered paternity. Child support orders were then pursued whether or not he was the biological father.

Here's another interesting fact I learned. After giving birth, a mother may decline to name the father on the birth certificate for several reasons. She may really not know who he is because she had multiple sex partners or the child was the result of a one-night stand. The father may be married and she may want to protect his infidelity.

Or sadly it could have been a case of rape or incest. In the state of Arizona, a woman cannot collect welfare, also known as AFDC, if she refuses to name the father. No exceptions are allowed. If a rape was involved, she would have to produce a police report. There are inheritance issues to consider as well. A child without the absent father on his birth certificate cannot collect the father's death benefits say from Social Security or Veteran's benefits. A woman gave birth in Arizona and declined to name the father on the birth certificate. He died shortly after the child was born. By law, that child could have collected the father's Social Security death benefits until his sixteenth birthday. Because the father was not on the birth certificate, the child had no legal standing. The mother was livid when she found out. She demanded to include his name on the birth certificate after the fact but it was too late. Hiring an attorney would make no difference.

A supervisor once let me sit in on an interview with a pregnant woman who applied for welfare benefits. The woman had just moved to Arizona from a Midwestern state. When asked for the father's name, she said she didn't know. She claimed to have impregnated herself after an exhaustive search of available men. She screened them for diseases such as HIV, hepatitis B, and other transmissible diseases.

"You just said you carefully screened out applicants," the supervisor said. "But you don't have the man's name?" She said she didn't. "Do you know where he lives?"

"Said he lived in a trailer park by my house," the applicant said.

"Why'd you move to Arizona?"

She just shrugged.

"To get benefits in our state you must name the father," the supervisor said. "Those are the rules. Come back if you can remember his name and address."

The dumbfounded woman and her five-year-old daughter walked out of the office. I stayed behind and discussed the case with the supervisor. In the past, a few women applied for welfare benefits claiming self-impregnation. DES calls it the turkey-baster method. An official with the department consulted several prominent obstetricians to determine if such a pregnancy could actually occur this way. All the doctors said the chances were about one in a million. Women claiming pregnancy through the turkey-baster method were denied benefits.

About a year later, I moved onto other volunteer work and left DES. During the time I was there, I felt like a valued member of the team. Employees treated me with respect and dignity. I was welcomed to the annual Christmas party. Staff members asked me to lunch. I admired their work ethic and how they got things done, with very little support from the state of Arizona.

Chapter Fourteen
The Sierra Club

In 2009, after leaving the Department of Economic Security, I searched around for another volunteer position to fill the gap. I enjoyed getting up in the morning with something meaningful to do. At the same time, my writing career had improved somewhat but not enough to get off Social Security. Advice I received at a few writing conferences suggested I look for an unfilled gap, a subject that others had not written about. I did just that and found my niche—animal shelters going green. In other words, replacing old facilities with energy efficient sustainable buildings. My research into sustainability was fascinating. I became so absorbed with a long list of innovations in the field that I pursued it further. I contributed about ten articles to animal and environmental magazines about sustainable animal shelters and even dog parks. Yes, dog parks go into the act. Not only did I learn about solar power, vegetative roofing, low-flush toilets, non-toxic paints, etc. but I met in person and talked on the phone to the most interesting people. For about two to three years, I attended monthly meetings of the Phoenix chapter of US Green Building Council, a leader in green building design and implementation. I rode the light rail to the downtown gathering place, reading a book or magazine on the way. I didn't like driving in midtown traffic plus I saved money on parking by using public transportation. As a disabled rider, I paid half fare.

Soon, I called the Sierra Club and started to volunteer for the Grand Canyon chapter in their downtown Phoenix office on a regular basis.

Sometimes, I took my rescued dog Dharma (now deceased) with me. Everyone on the office liked my dog and she soaked up the affection, especially the crunchy dog treats. On the way, we stopped at the Starbucks on seventh and McDowell for coffee. She was great company for the ride. At the Sierra Club, I did an assortment of office duties such as filing, shredding records, mailing, labeling, and whatever else was needed. Sometimes I arranged folders for important events like environmental day at the state capitol or other presentations. I called club members to invite them to the annual picnic. On their computers, I logged in information about weekend club hikes that took place at various public parks. Although I accepted my disability, I longed to go on these interesting hikes with fellow environmental lovers and sweat my way through a walk in the woods. I admired the chapter director and her assistant's tireless devotion to environmental causes—not just in Arizona but around the nation. Arizona's Republican-dominated legislature is often hostile to the wildlife and the environment, consistently voting against measures that guarantee protection for endangered animals or from the deleterious effects of mining or urban sprawl. The GOP is hesitant to chastise companies for bad behavior even when a river or stream is polluted from corporate carelessness. At every election cycle, the Grand Canyon chapter came up with a score card on legislator's voting records. Nearly all GOP members received a D or F grade. There was only one Republican in my memory, the late Senator Carolyn Allen, who received a passing grade. The GOP claims that environmental regulations stifle development. But don't they realize that clean air and water are harmful to the population? Even Republicans benefit from clean air and water and will be impacted by global warming.

In the early summer of 2014, I reluctantly left my volunteer position with the Sierra Club. For years, I had lived only about a fifteen-minute drive away. The rent on my trailer home increased every year to the point that I could no longer afford it. Reluctantly, I moved into a subsidized apartment building that was a much further drive away. I cut my ties with the Grand Canyon chapter but still pay my annual dues to the Sierra Club. I am proud that I contributed five years of service to the club.

Chapter Fifteen
Navigating at Sky Harbor Airport

In late summer of 2010, I called the public relations department of Sky Harbor airport to arrange an interview about the contraband sniffing Beagle (also known as the Beagle Brigade) in the Customs and Border Control Department. Two magazines were interested in the story. So was I. I had read about the Beagle Brigade in several animal magazines and how they worked at various entry points to the USA sniffing out contraband plants and food prohibited that passengers tried to bring in with their luggage, either inadvertently or on purpose. The Customs Department tried to rescue Beagles for this job, which impressed me.

I interviewed the border guard, toured the customs area, and met the Beagle, a rescued dog named Ranger that took his work quite seriously sniffing arriving foreign passengers and their luggage. That evening, the dog didn't find any contraband plants or food, but the guard said that in the past he made several important busts. Why are foreign plants not allowed in? Just one insect from a foreign plant can escape and start to reproduce. The result can be devastating and ruin crops with a loss of millions of dollars in damage. Foreign meats, even dried ones, can carry illnesses like Mad Cow disease. Upon entry to the USA passengers must declare what's in their luggage. The Beagle Brigade is added protection. Plus, it saves the lives of homeless Beagles.

Once my interview was over, I wandered around the airport for a while. I dislike flying but always loved airports. My dad drove us kids to La Guardia airport to watch planes take off and land on the observation deck. What a thrill.

On my night at the airport, I noticed an advertisement about the volunteer navigator program. I jotted down the number and called a few days later. That fall, I sat through a required one-day information class about airport operations then began a seven-week training period. I've been there ever since and these are examples of my experiences with passengers, employees, and visitors.

Airports around the US, including Sky Harbor, encourage passengers to arrive at least two hours before departure. Why? Traffic can be flowing smoothly when, suddenly, there's an accident or a stalled car that turns a highway into gridlock. Quick thinking cab or ride share drivers exit then head to the airport on side streets but that takes time, lots of time especially if you started out in Glendale or Maricopa, two cities at least twenty-five miles from Sky Harbor. Ticketing and baggage service can be unpredictable too. Airline management wants smooth service but glitches occur. Computer screens may suddenly freeze. Kiosks that dispense boarding passes may jam and not spit out a required boarding pass. Passengers may not have proper identification or balk at paying baggage fees. Lines at security back up if TSA employees call in sick or if there's a problem passenger, such as someone with a loaded gun. Yes, that really happens. Expect the unexpected but your experience at the airport will most likely be uneventful. And you won't miss your flight.

"May I help you?" I ask a passenger with the frazzled look as she exits the secured area.

"Where's the smoking area?"

"Take the escalator downstairs to level one," I say. "Exit to either the south or north curb and you'll find the designated smoking areas in the …" Wow, she's flying down the escalator before I finish. That was one of my earliest memories on my first shift alone as a navigator.

Nicotine-addicted passengers arriving after long flights, especially from foreign nations, are desperate to light up but Sky Harbor, like most American airports, bans indoor smoking. Several outdoor areas are set aside for smokers. Ash trays brimming with cigarette and the occasional cigar butts, particularly when wet, make my stomach churn. The nearby ground is often littered with ashes and butts as well. Smokers aren't the tidiest people. I know. I once smoked.

Volunteers rotate positions every shift. When I am stationed behind security, passengers frequently ask about smoking. There is no smoking inside the airport or any public building in the entire state. To satisfy those urgent cravings they must exit security and leave the building. Some shrug it off; others decide it's not worth another potentially long wait to pass through security again. I always ask about departure time. If a passenger doesn't have at least 90 minutes I advise against going outside. Passing through security can be a breeze or the wait can take over an hour. Airport security is unpredictable. Passengers sometimes miss flights because of smoking. Airlines have the right to slap on fees when passengers miss flights because of their own negligence.

One afternoon, I noticed an anxious man pacing outside security. Turns out he waited for his wife who ducked out between flights to light up. Evidently, only scant time existed between flights and they failed to make the connection because of her smoking. Livid, the husband yelled about her bad habits as they headed to the Southwest Airlines ticket counter to rebook a later flight. The wife acted contrite, trying to blow it off. If they hadn't been in such a busy public place, I imagine the argument would have been escalated. I hope it wouldn't have turned physical, certainly not over a cigarette. That would've prompted a call to the airport police.

Meeting and greeting passengers from around the US and all over the world is exciting, challenging, and fun. I usually see the best of people, but not always. In such a heavily traveled airport, passengers are often in a hurry. Some are impatient, chastising employees and volunteers for flight delays caused by weather or mechanical issues. Wallets with cash, electronics, passports, clothing, and other personal belongings may be left behind in airplanes, bathrooms, restaurants or outside in the dog park (yes, we have dog parks). Airport employees, visitors, and passengers turn in lost items, some quite valuable, to volunteers or airport personnel. My faith in humanity is restored by people's honesty. One day a passenger found a $100 bill and turned it in to me. Since it was for a large amount, I called airport police and turned the money over to the officer. An airport employee told me of a passenger who turned in a lost item. Inside was cash of over $7,000. Now that's incredible honesty to turn in that amount of money. If I find small change, I deposit the coins in the change box in the airport chapel where I often go to pray. After the COVID lockdown, the airport discontinued the donation box in the chapel. Now, if I find small sums of money, I donate it to the United Service Organization (USO). Once in a while, a passengers' lost items aren't returned. Presumably it has been kept by another passenger or even an airport employee or volunteer. If employees or volunteers are found with stolen property they are immediately let go.

All navigators are scheduled to work behind security every now and then. TSA is tasked with protecting us from harm, a tedious and stressful job. Constant vigilance is a must. Because my scooter cannot pass through the X-ray machine, a female agent screens me personally. Agents always explain the personal search procedure, especially around sensitive areas like the breasts because it is required by Federal law. During the procedure, I ask agents about their jobs.

A woman arrived at the security counter with a twenty-pound frozen turkey. Odd, I said to myself. What part of the country doesn't sell frozen turkeys?

"What'd you do?" I asked the agent as she performed her job.

"I ran it through the X-ray machine," she said. "The bird was clean so I let her go."

A search of a female passenger's upper body was halted when the agent felt a hard object. Agents escorted the woman to a private room where further investigation revealed the object in her bra. The finger sized glass vial contained a small amount of her deceased husband's ashes that she carried around as a source of comfort.

"What happened to the ashes?"

"Tested them for explosives. Came back negative so we let her go but not before recommending she pack them in her luggage next time."

Hoarders are often older women who collect animals, mostly stray dogs and cats. They live in filthy, overcrowded, and unsafe homes with stacks of newspapers and packages cluttering the hallways. A hoarder arrived at security. The gray-haired woman's blouse was filled with donuts, bread slices, and a corn muffin. Naturally, she was escorted to a private room. The food was removed and the security screening completed. TSA guards protect airports from terrorists. They are not counselors but this passenger would have benefited from a recommendation to seek psychotherapy. Hoarding is a sign of serious mental health issues.

Many years had passed since 9/11, that horrific day that changed America. I am still amazed that some passengers try to pass through security with weapons either strapped onto their bodies or in their carry-on luggage. A TSA guard stopped a US service man with a live grenade at a security checkpoint. I gasped just at the very idea of someone carrying a live grenade into any airport. Phoenix police removed the grenade. A live grenade, what was he thinking? I don't remember what the outcome was or how the grenade was disposed of.

Another TSA guard went out with friends after work for drinks. As she sipped a cold beer, she talked about her challenging job. She said passengers pack everything but the kitchen sink in their luggage then try to pass through security. The next day, a passenger actually arrived with a small kitchen sink. The guard cracked up. I did too.

There is a mail back program operated jointly by the airport and a UPS store just outside the airport. Items, mostly small pocket knives or tools that are not allowed through security, may be valuable or have sentimental worth to the passenger. Rather than dispose of them in the trash, which passengers often do, the mail back system was created. Passengers place banned items into a UPS envelope, fill out a contact form, and an airport employee slides the package into a safe. To participate, items must fit into the safe. A UPS store employee regularly empties the safe and then contacts the passenger to arrange for payment and delivery. The airport serves only as an intermediary.

One afternoon I started my shift at an information booth outside security. A Phoenix police officer escorted a smooth-talking woman in a snazzy gray and white pant suit to the counter. He asked about the mail back program for a stun gun. It's been years since 9/11. Who would try to pass through security with a taser? The elegant fifty-something woman in front of me, that's who. She talked to the police officer about the weapon as casually as if it was the latest cell phone. In front of me lay the stun gun, a potentially lethal weapon. Honestly, it was benign looking, sort of like an automatic garage opener. I was glad I didn't have to touch it.

At that time, volunteers did not handle mail backs so I called the office for immediate assistance. As the employee handled the transaction I listened to the breezy conversation between wonder woman and the police.

"I picked up two tasers at a flea market a few weeks ago," she said with a suggestive stare. "I mailed one to my daughter. You just never know." No, you don't, do you? The banter flowed back and forth until she eventually completed the form. "Is that all?" she asked.

"UPS will be in contact," the employee said.

The officer escorted her back to security and the airport employee finished the transaction. As I watched them disappear into the crowd, I shook my head. Did she really think she could pass through airline security with a stun gun?

Every day, TSA guards confront impatient passengers who resent the screening process. Everyone, including airport workers and volunteers, passes through security. Workers who escort passengers on wheelchairs might be screened seven or eight times a day. There are no exceptions. Even governors and senators must pass through security. Despite the abundance of stress, there is no room for rudeness. A small group of men, one dressed in traditional Sikh garb, approached me for help with TSA. I said wait here please, I'll find a supervisor. I motioned toward a waiting area outside security in Terminal 3 (before the renovations), not as busy as Terminal 4. The guard brushed me aside saying they have to wait, we're very busy as he glanced at the bearded and head covered men. They were not. In fact, he never offered to call a supervisor. Ashamed and embarrassed, I asked the men to be patient. A supervisor would help them.

About twenty minutes later, the group leader approached me and said they're not busy. "They're standing around talking," he said. "Is there anyone else I can talk to?" I said to let me check with the office. I obtained a main TSA telephone number but as soon as I returned the leader had walked to the other security gate and found an empathetic supervisor. I watched the interaction for several minutes as the supervisor read over the man's paperwork. I assumed he provided the correct information so I left. At the end of my shift, I reported the incident to our supervisor who wrote up a report. Will it change the TSA agent's bellicose behavior? I don't know but at least the incident was placed on record.

Airline ticketing offices (in Terminal 4) are located on level two. Passengers are dropped off there by friends and family, taxis, airport shuttle buses, or the rental car shuttle. One afternoon, I headed to the office on level two for my break in our office.

Sniffling, a young woman holding a small child stood next to a luggage cart by door twenty-seven, not a usual place for passenger pick up. That's on level one. I asked if she needed help. "Yes, I do," she said. "I'm confused, I'm lost, and I don't know what to do."

"Please tell me where should you be?" I asked.

"My grandma is picking me up," she said. "I can't find her."

"She's probably waiting for you downstairs on level one," I said. "Let's head there. Does she have a cell phone? We'll call for you."

Tearfully, she said, "Don't have the number."

"OK, we'll figure this out," I said guiding the young mom to the elevators.

"My baby is hungry," she said.

"Do you have food for him?"

"I think I have some left," she said.

"Let's see if grandma is downstairs so you can feed that baby of yours."

After leaving the elevator, a quick search of the east waiting area turned up empty. I suggested that her grandmother could be waiting at the west end or at the curbside. "First, let's look outside and see if she's there," I said.

By now, the young gal's tears dried up. She seemed confident in my ability to handle her crisis. I hoped I could locate her grandmother without a cell phone. In situations like this, however, cell phones are so helpful. On the south curb I waited as her eyes scanned up and down. She did not recognize her grandmother.

"There's still hope," I said. "Let's check the north curb."

No doubt she was exhausted after a long flight with a toddler. She was also frustrated, hungry, and anxious. What would happen if her grandmother wasn't at the airport? She didn't have her phone number and I wasn't sure what else we could do.

As soon as we exited the door and stood outside, a gray-haired woman rushed up to us. Frazzled grandma drove around the terminal several times because airport operations personnel wouldn't let her double park in front. She admitted leaving late then running into highway traffic. So far behind, she lacked the time to park and wait inside the terminal. Grandma hugged me for my assistance. That's part of being a volunteer. Relieved for a happy ending, I finally took my break.

Often, passengers visit the information booth for gate data if it's not listed on the airport screens. Usually it is posted, but now and then a flight is dropped off for technical reasons. Some passengers leave quickly while others stay and chat for a few minutes if we aren't busy or they're not in a rush. A middle-aged man was in Phoenix for his wife's family reunion. He smiled as he talked about the weekend.

"I can't believe how lucky I am," the man said with a cute, boyish grin. "I married a terrific woman with the most unbelievable family. They all love each other." Every reunion, family picnic, and holiday gathering he'd been to is warm, friendly and loving unlike the cold sterile family he came from.

"I'm so happy for you," I said. "Not every family is so close."

"Been married for ten years now," he said. "I'm in awe of their togetherness, their bond. I love it. Thanks for your help. I see my wife coming now. She was in the ladies' room."

That brief conversation sent me slumping. I did not come from a close family. Uplifting family stories make me smile but at the same time I feel cheated. Why didn't I have a warm, loving family? Why do I miss out on cheerful family reunions, lively 4th of July picnics, or joyous holiday dinners? That gap will probably remain unfilled.

Two international travelers on a breezy walk on level three approached me with an unusual request. One lady was Kenyan, the other from Hong Kong. Both were in Phoenix for business. They wanted to snap photos in front of a store or plaque that said Arizona or Phoenix. I said follow me please, I knew just the place. I directed them to the small Phoenix art museum which suited their needs perfectly. They were so pleased when I offered to take a joint photo. And was I honored when the Kenyan woman wanted a picture with me.

A couple of elderly women shuffled along in the baggage section appearing somewhat lost. I asked how I might help. They rode the city bus to meet one woman's daughter who had a layover in Phoenix. I asked the flight number then escorted them to the waiting area on level three. Since there was almost an hour before the flight arrived, I pointed out our food court where they might grab a bite to eat or a cup of coffee. Smiling, the mother held up a brown paper bag and said I made our lunch.

"I bet it's delicious too," I said. "When your daughter arrives, there are plenty of tables to sit down and share your meal in the food court."

"We'll sit here and rest until she arrives," Mom said.

"Enjoy your visit," I said before leaving.

"Haven't seen my daughter in a few years," Mom said. "I look forward to our brief time together." I bet she did.

Volunteers once in a while confront confused passengers. Allegiant Airlines is a good example. The low-cost carrier flies out of the Phoenix-Mesa Gateway airport, which is about thirty miles southeast of Sky Harbor. Passengers who book connecting flights on Allegiant may not read the fine print on their tickets or travel itineraries. Upon landing, they ask where is Allegiant? The airline now has a small presence at Sky Harbor but most Allegiant flights are out of the Mesa airport. Many passengers respond with jaw-dropping stares to learn that it's at another airport not even close to Sky Harbor. A taxi ride to Gateway may cost at least $70 or more, depending on traffic. Van service is not available. Disgruntled passengers grumble about the fees but there is nothing we can do except to assist them with ground transportation to reach Gateway. I once overheard a woman screaming at her male partner that his stupid ideas didn't save them money after all. The moral to the story is always read the fine print when making travel plans so there are no surprises upon reaching your destination.

I was privileged to witness love, kindness, and compassion one afternoon. A husband and father waited for his wife to arrive along with their three children. Each girl held a special present for Mom—a bouquet of flowers, a box of candy, and a stuffed animal. Bunched together, the adorable girls watched the flow of passengers exit the secured area, standing on their toes with wide eyes to search for their mother. Dad stood close by obviously proud of his children, waiting also for his wife's return. What a valuable lesson that father imparted to his girls. Who knows, maybe he'd done it before. Respect for women was a value he held dear. The information counter was busy and I never saw the joyous family reunion. I am sorry I missed it.

I ran into three Latin ladies on level two near an elevator. Their English skills were as weak as my Spanish. I studied Spanish for eleven years in grammar school, high school, and college. I need practice to improve my fluency but I understand the basics. I directed the women to the ticketing section of US Air, now American, and continued on my way. Later on, I ran into the bewildered looking trio, boarding passes in hand. I guessed they wanted departures on level three. I said in my broken Spanish to follow me and left them at the security entrance. One of the women attempted to tip me with a few dollars and I signaled no. I said gratis, which in Spanish means free. Volunteers are not allowed to accept tips. All three smiled then we shared a group hug. After our warm embrace there were even bigger smiles. I waved goodbye. I was sorry I couldn't communicate more effectively. I vowed that I would improve my Spanish language skills since I already had a solid grasp on the basics.

Over the years I've volunteered at the airport, I've met hundreds of excited people waiting for friends and family. Some arrive with specially made signs that say *welcome home* while others hold flowers, stuffed animals, and candy yet others cry with delight when seeing their loved ones maybe for the first time in years. Death, illness, and other crushing reasons also bring people to the airport. I met a woman near the up escalator with a baleful look. I asked if she needed help.

"On the way home for my mother's funeral," she said, glancing down at the floor. "I was just there for weeks and came home to be with my own family. Got the call that she passed away yesterday." Tears streamed down her face.

"I'm so sorry," I said. I lifted myself up from my chair and hugged her.

The red-faced woman said, "Thanks. I'll be OK."

"Are you sure?"

"Yes, thank you."

And then she was on the escalator headed to the departure level. She seemed so fragile, feelings so easily broken. A supportive family waited for her. That's more than most people have including me. I was truly sorry for her loss.

The airport embarked on a restaurant construction phase in 2012. Older restaurants closed and new ones opened. The Phoenix City Council offered local restaurants the chance to open eateries in the airport. Le Grande Orange, with a restaurant in central Phoenix, scheduled their grand opening in late October. To build up an airport clientele, the restaurant manager handed out dozens of free invitations to airport employees and volunteers. I received one and said why not try out the free offer. Only employees and volunteers with invitations were allowed in that afternoon, the day before the grand opening. The restaurant pulsed with loud music, hungry people, and an exciting atmosphere. I ordered a vegetarian pizza that I took with me since

I was still on duty. That pizza was one of the tastiest I'd ever eaten. The crust was scrumptious, the vegetables fresh, and the sauce sweet and tasty. If passengers ask what's good in the D gates I always say Le Grande Orange. I was a very satisfied customer.

Children are often in the airport both as travelers and as visitors, with their parents or guardians. Seeing a child, about four or five years old, walking through the food court alone one day shouting, "Papa, papa," caught my attention right away. I asked the boy about his papa. He shrugged as if he didn't know. I said come with me and we'll find your papa. Over the years I'd encountered lost bags, lost cell phones, lost books, etc. but never lost children. I said to myself, if we don't find papa by the time we reach the information counter we'll call airport police. This was serious. I told the boy to let me know as soon as he saw papa. About two minutes later, a gray-haired man barreled up the escalator stairs into the food court. Sweat poured down his face. The little boy let go of my hand and started to run toward the man. "Papa, papa." I followed him in my chair. The older man, who was his grandfather, was in the men's room when the boy suddenly ran out. Since his pants were down, it took him a few minutes to compose himself then run after his grandson. He was grateful I found him. So was I.

Passengers approach the information desk with all kinds of questions, most of which are routine and flight related. A man asked about boarding passes. I pointed out the kiosk where he could print a boarding pass since he traveled without luggage. He frowned then said, "You mean I have to print it?" Spoiled, wasn't he?

"The other alternative," I said, "is to wait online in ticketing on level two."

"No one is here to print my pass?"

"No sir, not here, just on level two."

He shrugged. "My wife usually does this for me."

I wasn't sure what to say. "Sir, the kiosks are over there. They're user friendly."

He stormed away and eventually, aghast he had to print his own boarding pass. I wonder if he called his wife to complain the airport wouldn't print his boarding pass.

Don't judge a book by its cover. That lesson applied to me on my assignment in the baggage area. A group of young men with facial jewelry, tattoos, baggy jeans, and high-top sneakers asked me for directions. As always, I responded with a smile and answered the question. Not only were the guys warm and charming but they seemed concerned about my disability. One asked if I needed help. I laughed and said I'm here to help passengers like you. Honestly, I would not approach someone with extensive body tattoos or facial jewelry for casual conversation. Talking to these young men however reminded me that beauty is only skin deep. Judge someone by what's in their heart, not by how they look.

A man with thinning gray hair wearing pleated gray pants and a blue polo shirt hurried to the information table in baggage. He said I have a problem, please call the police. I asked what happened. He seemed in apparent distress and I hoped he wasn't ill.

"My car was stolen," he said.

"Where were you parked?"

"Outside on the curb,"

I rolled my eyes around. "For how long?"

"About an hour."

"Sir, your car has likely been towed. Curbside parking isn't allowed at this airport," I said. Curbside parking isn't allowed in any US airport. "We make frequent announcements that if you leave your car it'll be towed."

I called security and, sure enough, his car was towed. I directed him to the airport bus that would deliver him to the parking facility.

"How much will it cost?"

"Not sure," I said. "The police will tell you but there is a fine. They accept credit cards." From what I knew of towed cars and fines, I suspect the man's bill would likely be closed to $200, much less than if he had parked his car. The airport also provides three free cell phone lots where family and/or friends can wait, for free, in their cars until passengers arrive.

If passengers or visitors have trouble locating their cars, which sometimes happens, an employee from Ace Parking, the company that manages airport parking services, will drive them around until they locate their car. The service is free and I recommend it to passengers who are unable to find their cars. I've used it too! As a rule, I always park on level five in the same area. A few times level five was full so I had to park on level six. I once forgot that I had parked in another spot. Frustrated that I couldn't find my car, I reluctantly pushed the help button and summoned an employee who promptly found my car.

The airport is friendly to passengers traveling with pets. Dog parks are located outside each terminal, available for passengers and/or visitors with dogs. Airport police and customs dogs also use the parks. One morning, I entered Terminal 4 and passed an elderly man with a scraggly old dog on his lap. I smiled at the pair as I rolled by. The white-haired man grinned and asked for the time. His wife's plane wasn't due to arrive for another two hours.

"Jones and I got bored at home waiting," he said. "So we came here."

"Want flight information sir?"

"Nah, that's OK," he said. "Not in a rush, are we, Jones?" he said, glancing at his dog. "I miss my wife. Her sister is sick so she went to visit."

"Hope her sister is better," I said. "If there's anything we can do for you, please ask one of us volunteers. We all wear purple jackets."

During my shift, I later noticed the man reunited with his wife. The family exited the airport together; the old man seemed content. The tail wagging dog brought a smile to my face.

Airport employees fascinate me too. Each one has a unique past that I always enjoying hearing about. A ramp worker transferred from the Midwest to escape the brutal winters. Howling winds slapped him around handling baggage in sub-zero temperatures. Weather so cold his feet felt like slabs of ice even with fur lined boots wasn't enough to stay warm. Finally he applied for a transfer to the Southwest and landed in Phoenix. Even our triple digit summer weather doesn't bother him. He's glad to have a job especially away from the icy cold winters.

Immigrants from Somalia, Egypt, Nepal, Mexico, Liberia, and other developing nations work in the restaurants, maintenance, and as wheelchair escorts. Many arrived in the US as refugees, fleeing from harsh unstable regimes. One Somali woman I talked with only remembers a nation ripped apart by war. There was no period of stability in her village, just warlords, guns, rape, and destruction. She jumped at the chance to leave, although she misses her family. We've become friends. I visit her family regularly especially now that she left her airport job to have a baby. Others from the Sudan and Congo share similar tales of death and destruction. I feel fortunate to live in the US and so do these refugees. In fact, my Somali friend, Qamar, invited me to her citizenship swearing in ceremony in 2013. I was honored. Normally quiet and reserved around strangers, Qamar spoke in front of the audience of hundreds saying how honored she was to become an American citizen. She said how much she loved the US.

For thirty-five years, I called New York City home. I could sit for hours in a café or restaurant and watch people as they walked up and down Broadway. The airport is another thrilling place to people watch. It's easy to spot late passengers because they race through the airport trying to reach their gates on time. I always cheer for them, hoping they make their flights. Foreign passengers, curious about Arizona, snap pictures, and buy mementos to take back home. I hope they enjoyed their stay. Family travel plans can fall apart if there's a weather delay. Waiting for hours with cranky toddlers inside an airport tugs at parent's nerves. Naturally passengers just want to go home. I hope stormy weather clears so the planes can take off and land soon.

In April 2013, the Phoenix Sky Train opened an automated tram that connects Terminal 4 (the busiest) with east economy parking lot, the light rail station and Terminal 3 (November 2014). On my first shift at the light rail station, I met a middle-aged man who needed help. He said stations like this make him nervous and needed help to the platform. I rode my scooter next to him. He asked if he could hold my hand. He walked next to my scooter, holding my hand. I sensed that he was really uncomfortable. I rode with him on the elevator to the platform to wait for the train. I asked if he wanted my company to the security gate. He said no that he'd be OK. I suggested he look for other navigators in Terminal 4 if he needed more assistance. My job as a volunteer is not to judge people but to assist them.

On that same shift at the light rail station, I met the most awesome group of people. They were organizers for a spiritual conference scheduled for the weekend at Arizona State University in nearby Tempe. Students and young adults from around the US and Canada were expected to arrive throughout the day. Nearly all were Hindu's of Indian descent but the spokesman said religion or race did not matter. The conference was about teaching leadership skills, values, and kindness. I shared those same beliefs and for a few brief moments we talked about spreading joy in the world. The conference leaders were very well organized and I expected that the participants left with valuable messages to embrace in their personal lives. Meeting those people uplifted me. I left with feelings of hope.

One day, I noticed a man with snowy white hair shuffling along level two, the floor for ticketing and check in. I rode my scooter next to him and asked if he was leaving on a flight. Yes, he was. I suggested a wheelchair escort since he had trouble walking. Each airline employs a wheelchair escort service. Workers push passengers with mobility issues directly to their gates. The older man said that sounds like a good idea.

"American Airlines escort service is just ahead." On the way I asked him where he was headed.

"I'm sixty-eight years old and getting married," he said with a beaming smile. "I still have love and life left in me."

I smiled as well. "Sir, I wish you and your new wife all the best."

I left him in the very capable hands of the escort service that promptly seated him in a wheelchair and headed toward the elevator. That made my day. Maybe one day I'll be able to say the same thing—that I'm getting married.

At the information station a frazzled looking mother appeared holding a little boy's hand. On the short Sky Train ride from the east economy parking lot to Terminal 4, the little boy left his raggedy doll on the train. That was his safety net. Mom asked if we could call lost and found. I doubted that lost and found would have the doll on such short notice. The boy's pitiful look reached deep into my heart and I said to myself, we have to show this boy we care about his misplaced doll. I asked the employee to call operations, the department responsible for picking up lost items from information stations, knowing they would not have the doll in such a short time. Only a few minutes had elapsed since mother and son exited the Sky Train. But a simple telephone call would at least demonstrate care and concern. Then out of nowhere it seemed a passenger shows up holding a ratty looking doll. Could she have overheard the boy's desperate pleas to find his doll? The boy's eyes glowed and his mother hugged the unknown woman. I was so thankful that a stranger, perhaps a mother and grandmother, saw the doll and realized it may have significance to some child. What a gift for me as well as mother and son.

On an evening shift, I was posted outside of the international area. The once daily London flight had recently arrived. That flight brings hundreds of passengers from all over Europe, Asia, and Africa. I noticed a group of women, all in floor length black dresses, including head coverings. I assumed they were Muslims from Saudi Arabia, having made the connection to Phoenix in London. Bewildered faces suggested they were lost. I rode over on my scooter to see if I could help. That's when I noticed crosses hanging from their necks. I realized they were Christians, not that it mattered. They needed help, regardless of religion, race, or ethnicity. Turns out they were Greek nuns here to visit a monastery outside of Florence that I didn't know existed. One or two of the sisters spoke passable English and presented me with a local phone number. I called and a man said he'd meet them in fifteen minutes by door four in baggage. I escorted the nuns, waiting until their driver arrived. The man and several assistants arrived promptly, bowing to the nuns. They loaded their guests and baggage onto a van. The nuns thanked me for my assistance. I hope their time in Arizona was special.

Another day, I was posted behind security. The information desk is at a place we call the high B gates. There was a lull in incoming flights so I took a break. I wandered around for a few minutes to check out the newly opened restaurants. On my way back, I passed a man who looked familiar. I kept rolling but I couldn't shake that face. Then it hit me. That was Mark Kelly, now AZ Senator Kelly, the retired astronaut, and former Congresswoman Gabby Giffords husband. The woman in a wheelchair must be Giffords. So I turned around and approached them. Former US Congresswoman Gifford was severely injured in a shooting at a public event in her Tucson district on January 8, 2011. The gunman, Jared Loughner, opened fire on Giffords and turned his weapon randomly on the crowd. Eighteen people, including Giffords, were shot; six died including a nine-year-old girl.

"Excuse me," I said. "Hello, we've met before. I volunteered for Janet Napolitano when she was governor and I met you at a fundraiser."

Both Giffords and her husband smiled. I wanted to be quick because they were obviously on the way to catch a flight. I surmise they didn't want to attract attention either. In addition to her position as a former Arizona legislator, Giffords and her husband were now involved in national gun control efforts. They were well known throughout the state and the country.

"I'm very sorry for what happened," I said, referring to that horrific day in January 2011. "I have a brain injury too but mine was caused by a car accident. I volunteer here at the airport. I wish you all the best. It was nice meeting you."

Giffords again smiled and Kelly said thank you. Due to the severity of Giffords brain damage, her speech is impaired. And then they were gone. I felt honored to meet them. I am truly sorry that her political career ended as a result of violence rather than an election. The accident changed my life. She was injured far more severely than me. I hope she continues to make a difference in her second life.

Phoenix scored big by landing the Super Bowl, footballs game of games in 2015 and again in 2023. Actually, the football stadium is in Glendale, a city that hugs the northwest edge of Phoenix. Months before the annual game, the city spruced itself up in preparation for the onslaught of visitors from around the country. The economic impact was worth millions with visitors expected to open their wallets for hotel rooms, rental cars, food, alcohol, souvenirs, and much more. Airport volunteers were ready too. Supervisors asked volunteers like me to work extra shifts before and after the Super Bowl to handle the extra passengers expected to flood the airport. I signed up to work two extra shifts. On one such shift in 2015, a middle-aged man with a slight grin approached me and asked,

"Any chance of you arranging a private meeting with Katy Perry?" pop singer Katy Perry was the lead act during the gala intermission half-time show.

I laughed to myself. "Sir, there's a lot of things I can do here at the airport but that's not one of them."

"Didn't think so but I thought I'd ask."

"Have a good day," I said, grinning.

On my second Super Bowl shift, again in 2015, a young man and his buddy, both dressed in jeans, T-shirts, and sneakers casually walked up to me. One of them said, "Hey lady, we'd like to get tickets for the game. Is there any way you can help?"

Again, I laughed to myself. "There's no way I can get tickets," I said. "Sorry I can't help you."

"Sold out, right?"

"That'd be my guess."

If I did come across an extra ticket, I'd have sold it on eBay or Craig's List to the highest bidder and used the proceeds to settle my debts and take a vacation. I could care less really about seeing the game in person. There'd be way too much noise, traffic, and chaos.

Lots of volunteers stepped up to work extra shifts during both Super Bowl games to ensure that airport operations ran smoothly and that our passenger's needs were met. No one received compensation, tickets to the game, or one-on-one meetings with the players. We chipped in because we're dedicated to the airport and we love serving the passengers of Sky Harbor.

Passenger questions are mostly about arrivals, airport services, parking, or food. Now and then a passenger comes up with a doozy. I call it California time and here's why. A passenger casually approaches the information table and asks me if I have arrival information about the flight from California, which is the most populous state in our nation. Dozens of flights arrive from California from such cities as San Diego, San Francisco, Los Angeles, Orange County, Bakersfield, Sacramento, Fresno, Palm Springs, Santa Ana, Oakland, San Luis Obispo, and San Jose. "What city please?" I ask the passenger.

"Don't know."

OK, I can tell this won't be easy. "The airline?"

"Nope."

I suck up my frustration and smile. "Where does the person live?" hoping that will narrow down the choices of arrival.

"Not sure."

"There's no way I can help you." I remind the passenger that California large with dozens of arriving flights on United, Delta, US Airways, and Southwest. United and Delta are is in Terminal 3 and Southwest/US Airways are in Terminal 4. "Does the person you're meeting have a cell phone?" If they do, I suggest waiting for the person to arrive. "Let them call you and ask where they are. That'll help you find them."

If the passenger doesn't have a phone, I suggest waiting around for a little while then using the paging assistance location, also known as PAL. The PAL has since been discontinued. It sent out an announcement throughout the terminal that I hope the missing passenger will hear. Now, we page the person on the airport announcing system. California time requests are so unsettling to me as well as other volunteers. There's only so much we can do to assist a passenger with so limited arrival information. Such questions have been posed to other volunteers too.

There is an information table the high B gates. The A and B gates serve American and the international airlines. If a shift is adequately staffed, a volunteer is assigned at the high B gates. We answer questions mostly around food. For example, a passenger may ask for a recommendation for vegetarian or Mexican themed food. Or if it's football season, passengers, ask for a bar to view the game and have a drink. Some just want a sandwich and coffee. Now and then a passenger asks about transferring to another terminal, how to catch a taxi, or the rental car center. One day a dapper, clean shaven, middle-aged man posed an unusual question.

"Any place in the airport where I might buy a new suit?"

"Honestly, sir, no there is not," I said, wondering why he needed a new suit. He seemed perfectly dressed to me in casual attire of neatly pressed khaki trousers, a blue cardigan, and an open neck pullover. Now, there are at least two men's clothing stores.

"I have an important meeting tomorrow morning," Mr. Manners said. "The airline lost my luggage and I'm desperate for something more suitable to wear than what I have on." He seemed ashamed, embarrassed.

"Only place I can think of is the Pro Shop," I said, nodding ahead of me. "They sell golf clothing. Maybe they'll have something suitable." I directed him to the store, only a few corridors away. I sensed he was a man of impeccable taste who was always on time, wore a suit and tie to work every day, and had his shoes shined regularly. Showing up to meet with colleagues in casual attire would perhaps humiliate him. I hoped his luggage either caught up to him or he found proper attire for his meeting.

A young Spanish speaking couple asked for directions. I managed to cough up a few Spanish words to properly answer their question. As I glanced down at the girl, about seven or eight years old with them, my heart sank. I choked back tears. The girl's body was scarred, apparently with burn marks from a fire. I reached into my bag of small rubber airplanes and held them out in front of the girl. She chose a pink one.

"*Muy bonita*, very pretty," I said as the disfigured girl smiled at me with big brown eyes.

"*Me gusta* pink," I couldn't remember the Spanish word for pink.

She smiled again knowing that I liked pink too.

As the family got ready to walk away, I said *adios, tenga cuidado.* "*Tu es muy bonita*, you are very pretty."

I then rolled my chair into the nearby chapel and wept. I have no idea how she was burned. Maybe she was in a serious car accident like me. I'll never know. I prayed for the girl and the loving family who surrounded her. Alone in the chapel, I believed God brought me to the airport that day for a reason. As much as I complained about moving out of the trailer park where I had enjoyed living for four years and moving into a subsidized building in a neighborhood that I detest, I am still more fortunate than others. At least I have a place to live.

I ran into a female passenger in the baggage area, located on level one. All ground transportation services can be accessed there. The middle-aged woman asked me about taxis. Since we had recently added taxi's to both the south and the north curbs, I asked her where she was headed. Her destination? Payson! That;s about 90 miles north of Phoenix, in Yavapai County, and at least an hour and a half by car. I sincerely doubted that a taxi would even take her because of the distance.

"Payson is too far from here to grab a taxi," I said. "I'll show you the city-to-city shuttle. They have service to cities outside of Phoenix. They'll help you."

I escorted the woman to their desk and to my surprise the city-to-city shuttle did not serve Payson. In the almost five years I'd volunteered at the airport, I always assumed the city-to-city shuttle served Payson since it's a popular tourist destination. An employee, however, did provide me with a phone number to another shuttle that served Payson. I handed it to the passenger who made the call on her cell phone. The woman said she met a man online and flew to Phoenix to meet him. Evidently he never told her that Payson wasn't even close to the airport. I hope the woman's encounter with her newfound date turned out safe.

Passengers, airline employees, and guests of the airport sometimes misplace personal belongings. They may be in a rush to catch a flight or may be eating lunch and forget the carry-on bag sitting on the floor by their feet. Misplaced or lost items may be paperback books, sweaters, or shaving kits. I guess the man who left his shaving gear behind arrived at his destination clean shaven but without his razor and shaving cream. Other lost possessions are more valuable such as cell phones, purses, wallets, laptops, and prescription medicine. A bag of insulin can be critical to a diabetic passenger. Left behind items are picked up by good Samaritans throughout the airport in a variety of places including the Sky Train, bathrooms, security checkpoints, under airline seats, near the taxi stands, and in the food court just to name a few. Airport employees record each and every item handed in. Wallets or purses with cash over $100 are reported to the Phoenix police who handle them separately. There are three levels of airport lost and found depending on where an item was lost. TSA handles all items left at security checkpoints. Each airline has a lost and found system. And, finally, there is airport lost and found for items found throughout the airport in all three terminals including the rental car center, Sky Train and parking garages. The lost and found department is located in a small building nestled behind the operations center near the old Terminal 2. Terminal 2 closed down and all airlines moved to the newly renovated Terminal 3. Items are logged in by date and where they are found. So for example, if a passenger calls and asks about a missing cell phone, they would be asked to describe what the phone looks like and where they lost it to ensure a proper match. Some items can easily be identified, such as driver's licenses, and the passenger is notified by mail. In other cases, an identification can be made by telephone. All items are held a certain amount of time. After that, some are donated to charity such as clothing and books, others destroyed such as unclaimed cell phones or passports.

As a volunteer, it is always personally rewarding to assist a passenger to the lost and found to recover a lost item, particularly one of significance. A man I escorted to the lost and found was shocked to receive a message that someone had turned in his wallet full of cash. He had over $500 inside and the good Samaritan took nothing and instead returned the wallet to airport lost and found. Most people are amazingly honest.

Now and then I'll come across a passenger who loses a valuable item and it never turns up in lost and found but those cases are rare. Honesty prevails and that warms my heart and soul.

Travelers with disabilities are a common sight in the airport. Some are blind, led by service dogs or in wheelchairs. Escorts, if requested, accompany disabled passengers to the gate. One day on assignment at an information counter, I noticed a woman walking briskly toward a security checkpoint. The woman had no arms but her shoulders boasted colorful tattoos. I take for granted all my activities of daily living involving hands and arms, giving little thought to what I'd do without these limbs.

Appearance to me is everything. At the airport, volunteers wear purple jackets, polo shirts and casual slacks, skirts, or in some cases shorts. Management requires us to use good taste and to always be neatly groomed. It's a free country so passengers wear whatever they want. On any given shift, I may see a man wearing a tasteful suit, starched shirt, hankie tucked in his breast pocket and shiny black shoes. Alternately, I may see a man with a big hairy gut flapping out from under a wrinkled T-shirt. A woman's breasts popped out of her blouse one night as she ran to catch a flight. She must've felt the errant boob as it slid out of her low-cut blouse and quickly put it back in its place. Some look as if they took hours to get ready. Every hair is in place, there's not a wrinkle on the attire while others seem as if they dragged themselves out of bed, hopped in a cab and rushed to the airport. People watching at the airport is fun. I also go home thankful that I care about myself and how I look when I leave the house every day, even if most of my clothes come from a thrift shop.

The USO is a refuge at the airport for active duty and retired military men and women as well as their families. Open seven days a week from eight a.m. to eight p.m. (longer during holiday times), the USO offers light refreshments, a comfortable place to relax, and a play area for the children while military members travel. Televisions are available in addition to magazines, books, and reclining chairs. All services are free, courtesy of the airport. Many airports across the US have USOs.

During my time at Sky Harbor, I've either directed or accompanied service men and women to the USO. It is my privilege. Although I disagree with war, especially the invasion of Iraq, enlisted personnel do not have a choice but to fight. OK, I've read stories about soldiers who have raped women, even our own, in foreign countries, but the vast majority of service people are undoubtedly decent human beings. It's not for me to judge their character but to treat them with respect and dignity. That's how almost all soldiers treat me. Nearly everyone refers to me as "ma'am." Soldiers are always groomed and well dressed, even if out of uniform. Men act like gentlemen and women behave like ladies. My heart aches for the soldiers disabled from roadside bombs in Iraq/Afghanistan or wherever. I too have a traumatic brain injury and have difficulty ambulating. My mind is prone to confusion. At times, the pain inside my head pounds like a jackhammer. But my injuries were caused by a careless car driver not in a merciless war that never should've been started. I am sorry their bodies and their minds are shattered literally and figuratively. I hope we can prevent future wars so no one else has to endure the mind-numbing experiences of those war veterans. They served their country but their country didn't always serve them. I am pleased that at least Sky Harbor airport has a special place for them while they're on the road.

Since 1989, I've volunteered in animal shelters in several states. Of course I jumped right into the animal rescue scene as soon as I landed in Phoenix. Adopted pets are my favorites although I like all dogs and cats. I show kindness and mercy toward them all but shelter/rescue pets are especially dear to me. In Terminal 3 one day, I noticed a woman holding a kitten that she had just removed from a pet carrier. I presumed she'd just come off a flight and was giving the kitten some breathing space. Approaching the woman, I smiled and said we have a dog park outside but nothing for cats. She said the kitten just arrived from another state, an online purchase. I really didn't notice the breed nor did I care. I sucked in a whiff of patience and said have a nice day. Enjoy your new kitten. Hundreds of cats/kittens are available in Maricopa County shelters/rescue groups. They can also be procured online for free or little cost. It aggravates me that people shop online for live animals as if buying books on Amazon. There are also plenty of local purebred cat breeders. Online sales of purebred animals is, in my opinion, reckless, irresponsible, and adds to our already staggering problem of pet overpopulation. Since I was on duty, however, I said nothing, offering no admonishment. I am an avid supporter of rescued pets but at the same time I also value my volunteer role at the airport. It's not my place to lecture passengers about personal, political, economic, or social issues. I kept my big mouth shut although it was hard.

Unattended bags at Sky Harbor are a potential source of trouble as they are at airports, bus stations and in every public building. Most likely they were left behind by tired, careless passengers who just forgot about them. A bomb may be planted inside an unattended bag. Volunteers are instructed to call airport police immediately if we find one and never move an unattended bag. Jostling a suitcase with a bomb inside could potentially cause the device to explode. A police officer responds quickly to unattended bag calls and summons a bomb sniffing dog. If the dog clears the bag, the police officer removes the bag, inspects the contents, then takes it to lost and found. I've never witnessed the bomb sniffing dog detect explosives. In such a case, the police would declare an emergency and clear out the surrounding area. They would call for back-up. The city's bomb squad would be called to remove the explosive device. I imagine it would lead to chaos with flight delays, store closures, and a massive police presence. I hope that never happens.

What should I do, the woman holding a small dog asked? Assigned to an information counter in Terminal 4, I wondered what kind of evening it would be. Busy? Slow? I soon found out. An older woman, out of sorts, rushed up to our counter. Beside her stood a small wiry haired dog. She just arrived from Chicago, having parked her car in Terminal 2. Having stowed luggage in her unlocked car, she rummaged through her purse for keys. That's when her heart sank. There were no keys. Anyway, she asked, "What should I do?"

Gheesh, I said to myself, I'm not sure either. Frank, the employee on duty, asked a simple question. "Did you retrace your steps?" She had arrived from a flight in Terminal 4 but parked in Terminal 2.

"I really don't know where the keys might be. Could be in my son's apartment in Chicago or lost in O'Hare."

"Let me call operations to see if a set of keys were turned in recently," Frank said. None had.

"Is there anyone who has a spare set you can call?" I asked.

The passenger frowned. "I live in Pinetop."

Wow, what bad luck. That's several hours to the north.

"I only have one suggestion," Frank said. "Ride the elevator to level four. You'll see a blue kiosk. Press the help button for Ace Parking. Someone will meet you and maybe they can call a locksmith to help make a spare key."

The passenger left. We never saw or heard from her again. This passenger would have to pay for a locksmith but in view of the existing circumstances at least she'd get home.

The airport purchases small rubber airplanes that volunteers can hand out to children. Budgetary constraints only allow a certain amount of planes to be ordered annually so supervisors ask volunteers to dole out the planes sparingly. For example, do not give planes to adult passengers or to airport employees. They're strictly for children of passengers, especially if they're having a hard time. Special needs children appreciate the small gift. I offered a plane to an adorable little boy waited with his mom in the baggage area. Perhaps they waited for another relative or missing baggage. The boy, about four years old, dug his hand into my plastic bag and tried to take more than one plane. Eager children often do that when they see the array of colors—orange, blue, pink, yellow, and green. In a polite, friendly voice I say to the child that I could only give him one. "I have to keep the rest for other boys and girls like you." That wasn't the case with this little boy. His older brother, maybe six or seven, suddenly appears. He wanted an airplane for his brother. I felt like a heal.

"Hey buddy, you're trying to be kind and nice to your older brother and this crabby old lady says no, you can't have an extra plane. Do you forgive me?" I said.

He nodded yes. Mom winked approval.

I opened the bag. "Please, take another plane."

"Again, I'm sorry. I didn't realize your good intentions."

People in general can be thoughtless, careless, and inconsiderate. I see that behavior on every shift. The airport has carts available, for a fee, to help passengers ferry their luggage around the airport or to the parking garage. A person with manners would push it to the side so it doesn't impede foot traffic that includes parents pushing baby strollers, passengers in wheelchairs, or just people in a hurry. I've seen passengers remove their bags from a cart and just leave it in front of a busy escalator, elevator, or revolving door. As much as I'd like to admonish the person, I do not. Instead, I simply move the cart out of the way. Other people spit out bits of food in the elevator. They leave soda cans in the chapel. Dogs locked up in crates for long trips may naturally have to eliminate after arrival. I don't blame them for defecating in the airport but I hold their owners culpable for not cleaning up after them. Passengers spill soda, water, or coffee, and walk away, leaving a hazard for others behind them. Housekeeping is preoccupied with cleaning toilets, sweeping floors, and emptying out waste baskets. Responsible adults who cleaned up after themselves, their children, and pets could ease their burden. Rude thoughtless passengers however aren't the norm. Most people throw away their own waste, even dumping plastic bottles into the recycling bins. They'll alert an airport official to a spill or ask for paper towels to wipe it up themselves. If only everyone was on their best behavior.

I ran into a young woman in the baggage area once who was in tears. I wondered what was wrong? Had she just arrived home from a funeral? A divorce settlement? She passed right in front of me at the information table and I asked what was wrong. Evidently, the airline (I can't remember which one) damaged her suitcase in transit. That happens sometimes and we always refer them to the appropriate baggage office for a resolution. And that's just what I suggested. She continued to cry, showing me the damaged suitcase. Honestly, I've seen worse. The damage seemed minimal. She would file a claim and presumably the airline would offer her a settlement once she produced a receipt for the luggage. Her reaction seemed out of place. Perhaps something else was going on in her life. I didn't ask. I said I was sorry for her troubles and sincerely hoped that she resolved her luggage issue with the airline.

One evening, the food court was my assignment. Passengers are generally hungry, looking for a place to sit down and to eat. Most questions concern rest room location, parking, or baggage. I noticed a young woman with a toddler having a meltdown. The little girl was perhaps around four years old. Mom did her best to calm the hysterical child, kneeling down to her level and talking calmly to her. I rolled over and held out my plastic bag of souvenir airplanes.

"I have bad days too," I said. "Would an airplane make you feel better?"

The sad faced girl stopped crying and motioned that she wanted an airplane.

"Pick out your favorite color." She pointed to yellow. "Hope you feel better. You have a nice mommy who is trying to make you all better."

As I prepared to leave, Mom asked if her sister could have one.

"Would you like to pick one out for your sister?" I held the bag out to the little girl. Later on, I saw the family and the little girl was no longer in meltdown mode. Her face was full of smiles.

A gray-haired couple approached the information desk and also asked to use the phone. Sure, happy to help. They had just come from the London flight. The woman said her daughter waited in the cell phone lot. Where should they all meet? I asked what cell phone lot? The airport has three of them. The woman shrugged. Let me call your daughter. Please do, the woman said. My daughter probably doesn't know. She never comes to the airport. Sure enough, the daughter had no idea which of three cell phone lots she was parked in. It makes a difference. For example, if you are parked in the east cell phone lot you will land on the south side of Terminal 4. I will leave your parents on the south side near door eight. The daughter says I'll find them. OK, problem taken care of. The parents, who flew all the way from Tel Aviv, asked me to write down what level, what side, and what door number so they didn't get lost. I did as they asked. As I watched them walk away, I wondered if they would find the right door. I excused myself from my colleague, explaining the situation. I didn't find the couple outside so I presumed the daughter arrived. I swung around for one more look before heading upstairs and then I saw the woman, looking tense. Would I mind calling their daughter once more? Sure, no problem. The daughter was on the way. All was good or so I thought. On the elevator ride back to my post on level three, my phone rang. The daughter was lost. I described what I looked like and what I wore. Look for me outside door eight on the south side. When I exited the door, the couple was gone. I called the daughter. She finally found her parents. Another night at the airport ended safely.

On a routine Sunday afternoon, I answered a passenger's question. About what, I don't remember. The middle-aged woman asked if she could give me something. I hoped it wasn't an invitation to join a Jehovah's Witness church or something like that because I would have to respectfully decline. In the past, people have looked at my scooter, an obvious sign of a disability and assumed I'm in need of a miracle. They've handed me Christian prayer cards. Honestly, I've always been insulted. Don't assume because I'm disabled that I'm unhappy with my condition. Anyway, I responded affirmatively to the woman's offer which turned out to be quite a pleasant surprise. It was a small ceramic shaped, colorful flower with a small business card attached that said this is a Ben's Bell. Someone just gave this to you as a way to spread kindness. Please pass it along. I still have that small reminder of a stranger's awesome gesture of compassion. Maybe one day I'll pass it along to someone else but, in the meantime, it meant so much to me that I want to hold onto it.

A post in baggage suddenly changed from answering routine questions about the rental car shuttle and taxi's to angry shouting emanating from the nearby ladies' room. What the heck was going on? Before I had to chance to investigate, a police officer asked me to go inside and check out the situation. He waited right outside. I rolled my scooter inside and there stood a woman hurling vulgar insults into her cell phone at someone, maybe a relative, maybe a spouse, who knew? I motioned for her to keep it down. She did not. In walked the police officer and told the woman to stop yelling or he'd escort her out of the airport. At first, the angry snarling woman did not heed the officer's warning. When he didn't back down, she finally shut up. Meanwhile, I departed, leaving the matter in the police's hands. The loud mouth exited the bathroom along with the police officer. Later, she made another call but kept the tone at a tolerable level.

Stray animals have never been a problem at the airport. Passengers retrieve dogs that fly as cargo without problems. Most dogs and cats fly inside the cabin along with their owners. One day one of the employees noticed a rabbit poking its head out from the Global Entry office on the west end of level one. A rabbit? How on Earth did a wild rabbit find its way into the terminal? My colleague and I left out bits of lettuce for the little creature that we assumed was hungry. The rabbit gobbled up the lettuce right away. For about two days, the rabbit foiled attempts at capture until finally the airport rented a trap, the same kind used to ensnare feral cats. It worked like a dream. The rabbit was taken off the premises and let go back into the wild.

Volunteering at Sky Harbor was a challenge at first. I had trouble remembering that taxis were outside door seven on level one. The inter-terminal bus leaves from door twenty-two on level two. I kept cheat sheets on hand to look up what I couldn't remember. When I'm not sure, I ask employees. Now, after four years, I'm more confident but still ask if there's a question.

I love the excitement of the airport. No two days are ever alike. There is a song that says people make the world go round. People make the airport go round too. I'm glad to be part of the Sky Harbor community.

In March 2020, COVID curtailed air travel throughout most of the world. Our volunteer program closed down until August 2021. During that time, I missed my two weekly shifts. Staff at the airport kept us connected with Zoom meetings and emails. We were all glad to return after such a long absence. Not everyone returned. Perhaps they got involved in other volunteer work or they just enjoyed the time off. I couldn't wait to return. I missed the thrill of the airport as well as my colleagues. Serving as a volunteer gets me out of the house and connected to the world beyond my apartment.

Chapter Sixteen
Animal Rescue

In 1989, I started volunteering at the MSPCA, a private animal shelter in Boston. I volunteered in shelters in other cities and loved the experiences which ran from heartbreaking to exhilarating. I could write a separate book about all the experiences, good, bad, and indifferent. Not long after moving to Phoenix, I called the Maricopa County shelter and was put in touch with Barb Westermeyer, a short, wrinkled, wiry, chain-smoking woman who assumed many roles. Most importantly, she was totally devoted to her job. We bonded right away.

By mid-October, the extreme heat tapered off and Barb sprang into action for the off-site adoptions held at various locations around the county. The Mesa shelter was an old, decrepit, vermin infested building with rust, peeling paint and way too many animals packed into tiny cages. Too many people dreaded seeing animals in such deplorable conditions and often resisted visiting the shelter to adopt. Of all the animal shelters I'd seen, Maricopa County was by far the worst. I wondered why the county or the public wasn't ashamed of the deplorable conditions but apparently they weren't. To increase adoptions, the shelter brought animals to the public instead. Everything had to be transported to the sites including office supplies, pet food, bowls, animal crates, folding tables, chairs, as well as the dogs and cats available for adoption. Pulling off these events took massive planning. Barb was a master coordinator and I loved watching her in action.

"Darling," she called me one day. "I need you this weekend. Big event at Cave Creek Park. Can you be there?"

"What time and how to I get there?"

"Early," Barb said. "As for directions, heck I don't know. I've lived in Phoenix my whole life. I'm not good with directions. I'll ask my husband, Kenny, and call you back."

Barb offered a vague set of driving instructions. GPS wasn't available back neither and neither was MapQuest. The brain injury distorted what little sense of direction I had and naturally I botched my way to Cave Creek in northeast Phoenix. I lived in Tempe, located in the southeast part. About an hour late, I finally showed up at a gorgeous public park nestled in the sprawling desert.

"Sorry I'm late," I said as I rolled up in my scooter.

"Don't worry," Barb said. "Get ready to work. Ride back to the parking lot and look for the county truck. Pick up the stack of towels in the back. Dogs and cats need something soft to rest on while in the cages."

I spun around and located the pick-up truck Barb mentioned. In the back, there were piles of everything. I grabbed the linens and returned.

Patting me on the back she said, "I've got an important job for you." Barb's dedication to the shelter extended beyond her paid employment. In her spare time, she made gift baskets to benefit our unwanted dogs and cats. At off-site events, volunteers like me hawked raffle tickets. She plowed the proceeds into the foster care program so that tiny puppies and kittens born to moms that either died prematurely or had to be put down would find a second chance. "Sell as many as you can," Barb said.

Within a short time, I earned a place as one of Barb's top sales agents. I peddled raffle tickets at adoption events and raked in at least $200 at each one. And I loved it. The special part of the events, however, was the sight of dogs and cats on their way home with responsible loving owners. That made getting lost in unfamiliar neighborhoods worth my while.

•

On days off, Barb nudged local dairy farmers into donating goat milk for the foster care program. Puppies and kittens without moms had trouble growing on artificial breast milk. The young ones thrived on goat milk for reasons I didn't understand. The county couldn't afford the pricey goat milk so Barb's relationship with the farmers was crucial to the little one's survival. A freezer in Barb's office was always packed with containers of goat milk that volunteers caring for puppies and kittens helped themselves to.

Even Barb's family chipped into her lifesaving missions. At off-site adoptions, Kenny helped out in whatever ways he was needed, mostly hauling supplies, or buying her a hot dog lavished with mustard and relish for lunch. Her mom brought her portable organ and played music. Sometimes her niece sold raffle tickets. It was like a family affair.

•

The cumbersome process of lugging crates, bowls, office supplies, chairs, tables, food, water, etc. to the adoption events ended in 2000 when PetSmart Charities donated a huge chunk of money for a mobile adoption van. We called it the Scratch and Sniff Mobile. Not only was the brightly painted van (more like the size of a bus) equipped with cages, a bathroom, and ample room for supplies, but it was air-conditioned. It was also huge. What a sight to see tiny Barb driving that big vehicle around. The Scratch and Sniff Mobile cut down on turnaround time to get to and from the adoption events and made transporting the animals a cinch. PetSmart Charities deserved all the credit.

•

As a regular shelter volunteer, I dealt with thoughtless owners and comforted abused dogs and cats. I watched dogs tug on their leashes after owners who surrendered them, saying the dog was too much of a bother. I saw the most despicable cases of animal cruelty, such as cats shot with arrows and dogs nearly starved to death. I cried as I saw tail wagging dogs or purring cats led to the back room, the end of the line, because the shelter neither had the space nor the resources to help them all. I grabbed the chance to volunteer for Pet Photos with Santa not long after I moved to Phoenix. I wanted to surround myself with people whose pets were cherished, beloved parts of the family.

PetSmart stores partnered with the rescue community for the three-week period before Christmas—Saturday and Sunday only. Each store provided the camera, frame, and film then split the proceeds with the rescue groups. Now, everything is done with digital cameras. I miss the days of watching the color photos pop out of the Polaroid cameras and then placing them into an envelope along with a holiday-themed frame, courtesy of PetSmart. Some pet owners were so pleased with their pet's photos they paid for seconds. High tech often saves money and time but it takes away part of the tradition too.

Sitting came easily to me because I had limited mobility from a pedestrian car accident in 1994. So, I wore the Santa suit, also courtesy of PetSmart. What a ball I had, even though the beard and the wig were itchy like a crinoline slip. Some big dogs were terrified of having their pictures taken with me dressed up as Santa. I struggled to hold them next to me. One giant dog was so scared he yanked me off the bench and started pulling me across the floor. Good thing I had a strong grip until the shocked owner intervened.

A fuzzball of a dog with a curly tail lifted his leg on my shoes and left me with a stinky memento. I shrugged it off as part of the job. A fluffy gray cat clawed my beard like it was a scratching post. One dog jumped in my lap and started to bark. A freckle-faced boy complained that I couldn't be Santa because I was a girl. After her dog's picture was done, one woman said, "I should've brought my horse. Maybe I'll come back." And she did. About an hour later, a woman riding a horse trotted across the strip mall and tried to enter the store. I watched with wide eyes as the bewildered horse was unsure what was happening. Management quickly derailed the horse owner's attempted entry.

Our gang of three—me as Santa, photographer, and assistant—headed outside to snap the pet photo with Santa. I stood next to the woman on her horse and smiled. Our photographer snapped a few photos. We went back inside the store then presented the woman, outside of course, with a choice of pictures. She handed me ten dollars, the charge for the pictures, which I then gave to the cashier. After each dog's photo shoot, we handed them a snack. We had nothing to offer the horse. That was one heck of an afternoon.

The sign in the store window said "Pet Photos with Santa." Most people showed up with dogs, a few with cats. Late one afternoon, a woman arrived with a small carrier. I assumed it held a cat, or maybe a rabbit. My mouth felt like chalk when I saw the large white rat. I grew up in New York City and to me, rats were unwanted guests. I would've screeched if I ever saw a rat of any color or size in my apartment. Fortunately, only the occasional mouse visited. Still, as Santa I had to act proper and pose with the white rat, even though I squirmed inside. I once posed with a pet chinchilla.

On bathroom breaks, I rode my scooter through the store. Customers called out, "Hey, Santa's on a scooter. Go Santa!" Some even applauded. I was pleased to see people's attitudes toward disabilities had softened.

A couple, perhaps in their mid-twenties, showed up one year with a turkey. The bird was well behaved and I posed with the bird, aptly named Tom. I had to ask how they acquired a turkey as a pet. The couple purchased the bird for Thanksgiving dinner. The bird stayed in their backyard for the few days prior to the big holiday. When it came time for slaughter, the husband chickened out. The husband said to his wife, "You do it."

She hedged and said, "No, I can't. You do it." The back and forth banter went on for a while until the couple decided against killing the turkey and bought a frozen one at the grocery store. They named the turkey Tom and kept him as a pet. When the husband noticed signs for pet photos, they said let's do it. And so they did. I was glad to oblige. I hope Tom had a long happy life.

One week during a pet photo session, a woman asked us an unusual question. She missed the Santa photo sessions at the nearby mall for her five-year-old son. Would we mind posing with him? Of course not. The little boy cuddled next to me and we took his picture. Hearing my female voice made him look twice but he still smiled and seemed satisfied. His mom paid the fee and left with her son's picture.

Over the years, I volunteered with many caring people from the rescue community. Some rescued dogs, others rescued cats and some rescued both. A few rescued horses. Everyone was dedicated to saving animals from abuse, neglect, and abandonment. A lot worked full-time jobs and had families. I remember a few times moms or dads with older children in tow at photo sessions. We adults handled the pictures and the children's presence just made it extra fun.

Pet owners who came for photos loved talking about their dogs and cats. I heard many stories about purebred dogs who competed in the show ring. Other people talked about pets they saved from unsafe situations or abusive owners. Take the middle-aged man who I noticed looking into the PetSmart grooming parlor one day. I said since you're having your dog groomed that maybe you'd like to have your dog photographed with Santa. The man said that was a good idea. He had been on a work detail in a remote part of the county and saw this haggard looking dog with his ribs showing. The man said he couldn't turn is back on the dog so he brought him home, had him checked out by a veterinarian and now to PetSmart for a much-needed grooming. I thanked him for his kindness. He later came to our little corner of the store where we took the photos and I gladly posed with this now spruced up dog that was in good hands. That made my day.

Every year I went home feeling warm and toasty about spending the day with people who adored their pets. It was worth all the time I spent stuffed inside a hot, scratchy suit just to see the human/animal bond at work. I needed days like that to renew my spirit. Otherwise, I wasn't sure I could return to the stressful conditions at the shelter. How many times could my heart break?

Pet Photos with Santa uplifted my spirts, renewed my commitment to animal rescue, and made me realize how many people truly love and adore their pets. I also appreciated PetSmart's commitment to animal rescue. Pets are part of our families. I loved my time also as a pet therapist. My life is fuller because of the experience.

·

Among the network of animal rescue people I met over the years was a woman named Julie Brown. Julie liked dachshunds, especially old, forlorn dogs without a chance for adoption. Sometimes she brought them home, tried to place them or prod a rescue to accept them. Now and then, she kept them herself.

One week, I bumped into Julie at the shelter. Two haggard looking dachshunds were impounded as strays. They also reeked, probably without proper bathing for months or even longer. Like most strays, the old gals came in without tags. What set one of the dogs apart was a huge tumor, about the size of a tennis ball that hung from her neck, nearly reaching the floor. Looking at the size of the tumor, it had to have grown for a long time. Didn't the owners notice? Without extensive testing, there was no way to diagnose it. The county's clinic only did spay or neuter operations and minor medical treatments.

"I feel so bad for those dogs," Julie said as she stared at the two old wiener dogs. "They had to be someone's pets."

"All of these cats and dogs belong to somebody," I said.

"No one will adopt these two. Maybe I can get someone to take them."

"That's a tall order for senior, sickly dogs, especially the one with the tumor," I said. "Tell someone in receiving that you're trying to help so they're not euthanized when their time is up."

Julie contacted Coast to Coast Dachshund Rescue, a non-profit group that rescues dachshunds from shelters or other unsafe situations. When possible, they arrange for transport across the country to either a foster home or a permanent arrangement. Some kind soul took in the old wieners. One lived about six months and other for around eight. The quality of their original home appeared to be lacking but at least the weenies enjoyed a few good months before expiring. I'll always remember how Julie went out of her way to help those two senior gals. We've been good friends ever since.

·

For months, friends and rescue colleagues talked about the local dog parks and the fun they had as their dogs frolicked in the enclosed spaces. In my dog Maxine's healthier days, she would've enjoyed a good romp around the grassy knoll but sadly she died in February 2001. On July 5, 2001, I made up my mind to visit the dog park closest to my home. After dark, of course, I brought my dogs, Luke and Judy. Just as I rolled my scooter toward the dog park, I noticed two stray dogs. Running after them was no longer possible. I watched the dogs as they scooted off. I asked a fellow dog lover if he would help capture the pair but the dogs proved elusive. Feeling sad and helpless, I took Judy and Luke inside and let them run around with the other dogs. Judy wasn't interested in playing and she sat next to me as I talked to other dog owners.

One of the stray dogs followed us to the parking lot. I opened the door and the black dog jumped in. Judy and Luke jostled with her in the back seat. If it wasn't for the late hour I would've driven the stray dog to the county animal shelter. They were closed at that time. Instead, I took her home. Almost entirely black, I assumed she was a lab mix. She was young and friendly. I checked her for ID but she had none. By the next morning, she had worked her way into my heart. I wasn't sure if I would keep her but I decided to find her a good home. Summertime was always hard to place adult dogs and cats so I ended up with another dog. I named her Midnight. She was the greatest dog and lived until the fall of 2013.

Over the years, other shelter dogs needed me. I brought home Dottie, a dachshund that had been used only to breed. When I got her, she was old, sad, and anti-social. But she learned to love Luke and spent a year and a half surrounded by love and affection.

Then there was Ziggy. She was old and blind. Ziggy's owners confined her to the yard and rarely bathed or brushed her. A groomer spruced up Ziggy for free so she'd looked pretty. No one wanted her because of her age and disability. I couldn't let her go so I took her. I also took home Fred, Dharma, Flash, Casey, Lucy, Oscar, Dolly, George, and Franny, all old unwanted dogs. Some lived a few weeks, others lived a few years. All of them enjoyed the comforts of home before they moved on to another life. As of this writing, I have Whitley, also adopted.

A stray dog delivered puppies in a city park. A good Samaritan tried to scoop the puppies and the mother dog into his car for transport to our shelter. In the process, the mother dog took a chunk out of the man's hand. The shelter quarantined the dog for ten days, standard practice with dogs and cats, without a rabies vaccination. Because Mom had an attitude, Barb had to find a foster home for the puppies. Mom wasn't trustworthy and would be euthanized at the end of the ten days. At the ninth hour, Barb scrambled for a place for the puppies.

"They're going down tomorrow along with the mother," she said with her head buried in her hands. "All our foster homes are busy. I feel bad for the little ones."

I hemmed and hawed. "I'll do it."

Barb jumped out of her chair and hugged me. "I'll start you off with a big jug of goat's milk. Call me when you need more. I have plenty on the west side."

Besides the goat's milk, I left with a used play pen and six newborn puppies. For the next few weeks, I bottle fed the pups about every six hours. Luke acted like a mother, except he didn't have the right parts. It didn't matter because the puppies warmed up to him anyway. Judy ignored the squirming pups. Except for feeding times, the puppies slept together in a mound. Around the third week, the pups played as a team for a few minutes after eating. Then they slept for hours. By the fourth week, they were ready for solid food. I fed them a combination of goat's milk, baby cereal, and dog food. I took them in the backyard after feeding to start early potty training. By the sixth week, they were ready to be spayed and neutered. And then I had to return them to the shelter for adoption. A lump the size of an egg clogged my throat. How could I return six adorable mixed breed puppies to a cold, hard cage to be adopted by strangers? At the time, the shelter had shaky criteria for adoption. I worried about the kind of homes they would end up in. Would they be chained outdoors? Would they be abused? Or would they be loved and adored? I didn't want to relinquish my babies but keeping them wasn't an option either. Fostering puppies was so emotionally wrenching I never did it again, not even for Barb.

I rolled my scooter into the receiving part of the shelter one morning. There were several cat cages there for overflow cats/kittens. Cats breed in the spring and shelters are often inundated with litters from May through September. Maricopa County Animal Care and Control was no different. Kitten season was winding down so most of the cages were empty. One cage was covered so I presumed the occupant was either injured or sick. I peeked inside to see if the cat needed food or clean bedding. Yikes, she was giving birth. Unlike women in labor who scream, yell, shriek and pant, mama cat looked at me and said, "Meow." She seemed to be in no discomfort whatsoever. Having never had children myself, I'm sure women would like childbirth to go as smoothly. When mama was finished—she delivered two tiny kittens— we moved her to a larger cage. Honestly, her babies looked like itty bitty mice. They were about the size of my thumb. The kittens cried when I picked them up.

"Not to worry, my little friskies," I said. "I'll give you back to mama. I'm only fixing you a comfy clean place to rest."

As soon as I returned them to mama, the feline family cuddled together. Our foster care coordinator sent them to a temporary home until the babies were old enough for adoption. I hoped that mama found a good home too. Kittens and puppies almost always found homes. Mama cats and dogs weren't always as lucky.

A tail wagging German shepherd mix with a lot of spunk came down with kennel cough. The big girl ended up on the euthanasia list because kennel cough is contagious and spreads to other dogs. With little or no resources to treat the animals and no isolation unit, David, the manager, placed the dog on the euthanasia list. He glanced at Jared, a kennel worker, as he stood outside the back room holding the doomed dog with a leash.

"Someone call Caron. See if she can take this dog," David said, throwing his big arms into the air.

Caron had been involved with rescue since the mid-1990s with a group known as Dial A Pet. She took dogs off the E-list and brought them for adoption at PetSmart or at off-site events. There, she screened applicants and sent the dogs and sometimes cats to new homes.

"Put the dog back in the cage," David said. "Wait till the end of the day and let's see if we hear from Caron."

Jared returned the dog. And we waited. By the time I left that day, Caron hadn't called. I feared the dog with the curable cough would be euthanized.

"Caron came after work," Jared said the next week when I came back. "That dog was within inches of losing her life."

"That was the closest I ever saw a dog get to the back room and get saved."

I preferred not knowing their fate so I usually never asked. I made an exception this time. At the next available chance, I asked David why he persisted in saving this dog while so many others were euthanized.

"I can't really say," David said. "Maybe I was just sick of killing dogs and cats that day. I just had to save one. That dog was it."

I hope the dog had a good life.

•

To combat pet overpopulation, the county raised private funds to offer free spay/neuter operations to the public. The first 100 people were served. Some people lined up at midnight and waited hours to have their pets altered. That was commitment.

I don't know how the shelter managed to spay/neuter 100 animals in that cramped clinic. There were only two operating tables. Cats recovered on long tables in the hallway outside the front office. Little dogs were put inside clinic cages. Bigger dogs came out of the anesthesia on the floor, of course, resting on blankets. For a change, there were lots of volunteers around. The washing machine and dryer churned out towels, linens, and surgical drapes all day long. So many people clogged the small space it was amazing no one stepped on any of the animals. Yet four times a year the county went through this ordeal and altered at least 100 dogs and cats for the public, for free. Reducing pet overpopulation was worth all the aggravation of working in such tight quarters. We all worked well together even if we bumped into each other now and then.

September 11, 2001 was a turning point for the US. Like most Americans, I will never forget when the first of two passenger jets slammed into the World Trade Center. I was blown away by the horrifying events that followed and devastated that so many people might be dead or injured. On the television, I watched the World Trade Center collapse into a huge mound of rubble, burning ash, soot, and twisted metal. Devastated, I spent the day at the animal shelter. I didn't know what else to do. I feared the US would plunge the world into a spiral of hatred and violence for decades to come. I was also sure that President Bush would lead us to war. As we all know, he did.

September 2001 also brought other crushing news. Barb was diagnosed with metastasized cancer in her shoulder and abdomen. In the four years I had known her, Barb cried just once about the loss of so many shelter animals. The day she broke the news about her fatal diagnosis, she cried. I sobbed too. I wasn't ready to lose my dear friend.

"Barb, I don't know what to say, except I'm sorry," I said, wiping away my tears.

"That's OK, darling," she said. "I'm going to fight. You know me, I'm a tough son of a bitch." That she was.

"Good, when are you starting chemo?"

"Not just chemo but radiation too. Next week is my first treatment."

"Still doing the off-sites?" I asked.

"Sure am. We have one coming up and I expect you to be there," she said.

"Of course I will," I said.

As devastated as I was about Barb's cancer, I wasn't surprised. She smoked two packs a day and survived on a junk food diet. How could she fight cancer on glazed donuts, hot dogs, and sugary iced tea?

.

Around Thanksgiving that same year, I met a man who came to search for his lost dog.

"Barney has been missing for months," he said. "But I still look. Always hope he'll be here."

"Don't give up. Sometimes dogs and cats show up a long time after they become lost," I said.

"I doubt I'll find him but I have hope. My whole family has been heartbroken over his loss."

"How'd the dog get out?" I asked.

"We had someone clean our pool. He inadvertently left the gate open."

I heard that story dozens of times. Repair men and women left gates open and curious dogs escaped. Those with tags, if caught, usually went home. Those without had a less certain fate.

"Take a look around and if you find your dog, you know what the routine is."

If a pet owner found his dog or cat, they had to pay the fine. If the dog didn't have a rabies vaccination, they had an additional fee for the shot. No laws existed about cats. They didn't need a license or a rabies shot to go home.

A few minutes later, the man blew through the door to the receiving area and ran up to me.

"He's here," he said. "I can't believe he's here."

"I'm so happy for you."

"Wait till I get home. My family will be so pleased. We'll have a happy Thanksgiving this year. And Barney will get a plate of turkey."

•

Those small acts encouraged me to go back. As I pulled out of the parking lot, I swore I'd never return. By the following week, my emotional wounds healed and of course I dove back for more sadness, aggravation, and human drama. I couldn't stay away. The animals needed me.

Visits to the animal shelter were anything but routine. I never knew what melodrama, human or four-footed, awaited me. As a volunteer, I wasn't supposed to tussle with customers about why they turned in pets. For a big mouthed New Yorker like me, that wasn't easy but I followed shelter policy. I was only human, however, and my resolve cracked now and then. I waltzed through the front lobby on a sizzling hot July day when I noticed a big dog with short fur covered in so many ticks the bugs were falling off the dog, landing on the floor. The dog looked like a cutlet, dipped in egg and breaded but with ticks instead. The bugs were scattered everywhere. Customers with large canines steered clear of the buggy mess. Owners clutched little dogs and cats in their arms.

"I hope you're here for a tick dip," I said. For many years, we maintained a huge pool of tick dip in receiving. Every impounded dog got a quick dip into the harsh chemicals to rid them of ticks. We offered tick baths to the public for ten dollars. The shelter now uses a less toxic treatment and just as reliable.

"Turning him in," the man said.

If I said something sarcastic, he might change his mind and storm out with the dog. That would place the dog in further harm so I shut up. I watched the clerk finish the transaction. The man walked the dog to receiving. The dog was immediately euthanized and put out of his misery. I hope that man never acquired another dog.

•

Another dog up for adoption, a sweet cocker spaniel, was also crawling with ticks. The flea dip obviously wasn't enough in her case. I took her outside and picked off the pesky bugs, one by one. Sandy, an older woman who volunteered for Arizona Basset Hound Rescue, noticed my futile effort.

"Here," Sandy said as she sat on the bench next to me. "Let me help."

As we both plucked ticks from the cocker, Sandy said, "I should call my brother, Don. He and his wife just lost their cocker a few months ago. Maybe they'll want to adopt this gal and give her the great home she deserves."

"A home without ticks, that is."

A few months later, I ran into Sandy at a dog park. Don and his wife adopted the tick infested cocker. They brought her to a groomer, had her treated for ticks, and made her the lady of the house. If I hadn't brought that dog outside to take off the ticks, Sandy wouldn't have noticed. She only came to the shelter to pick up a dog tag for Arizona Basset Hound Rescue. The flotilla of fate worked well that day.

·

Barb's health faded. Over the next several months, she was in and out of the hospital. I spent Christmas of 2001 at her hospital bedside because she was so sick. Barely able to work, another employee absorbed her job responsibilities, including the role of off-site adoption coordinator. That made Barb so sad but she just couldn't hack the full-time role. Of course, she was welcomed anytime at the shelter but others carried on in her place. The place wasn't the same without her.

The employee who took over the off-sites lacked Barb's pizzazz, insight and coordination skills. The events, in my opinion, weren't as lively or fun. And the new person didn't include the popular shot and licensing clinics that Barb had organized. On those days, we were so busy I spent hours writing dog licenses and rabies vaccination certificates. We filled the county coffers with thousands of dollars thanks to Barb's resourcefulness. Without her, the off-sites lost their luster. I may have attended a few but after a while, I stopped going. I offered suggestions on Barb's winning ways yet no one seemed interested. That turned me off.

One day, I was rolling through the shelter and a man, about thirty years old, taunted a pit bull impounded as a stray. The man's son, probably five or six, watched as his dad kicked and punched the dog's cage. The father had a wicked grin. I went ballistic. Instead of the helpful role I usually played, I turned into one tough broad.

"Stop that," I yelled. My heart pounded as I rose out of my chair and stood in the man's face. I flung my hand at the exit sign. "Get out."

The man looked incredulous.

"You heard me, get out," I said. "What kind of role model are you, assaulting a helpless dog in front of your son?"

"I was just …"

Sweat poured down my face. "I said out," pointing to the exit sign. "Go, now."

The man finally stormed away. Meanwhile, other customers heard the angry confrontation. They applauded after the monster was gone. "Good for you," a woman said. "I hate when people are mean to animals."

"He's gone now, but we can't prevent him from getting an animal. And who knows what kind of life his kids have?"

I told David, the supervisor, about the spat. He jumped out of his seat and said, "Where's the bastard? I'll throw him out if he's still on the premises."

"He's gone."

Other supervisors wouldn't have been so supportive, even though the customer had clearly violated shelter principles against animal mistreatment and common decency. I was so glad David was on board.

Scenes like that happened numerous times during my tenure with the county. David wasn't always around but each and every time I challenged visitors who teased and taunted the dogs, asking them to please stop. I refused to tolerate animal mistreatment in our shelter against dogs or cats.

A clinic worker, also named Deb, once said, "Aren't you afraid of these scum?"

"Absolutely not," I said. "I worry that other people sit back and say nothing. Violence against animals leads to violence against people. I can't change the world but I won't stand for it here or anywhere else."

"They see you're disabled. You might get hurt," Deb said, staring at my scooter.

"I'll mow them down with my chair and whack them with my cane."

We both cracked up. All kidding aside, animal cruelty was a serious offense that I didn't take it lightly. People who abused animals rarely stopped there.

•

By February 2002, disease had ravaged Barb's body. Her weight slid down to about eighty pounds. We kept in touch by phone at least every ten days. The end was soon and I had trouble facing reality.

I called one evening and her husband Kenny answered.

"Better get to the hospital soon," Kenny said. "I'm afraid she won't last much longer. She's barely conscious but I think she'll know who you are."

The lights in Barb's room were dimmed. Tubes, catheters, and breathing machines kept her alive. Her body looked like a skeleton as she lay on the bed hovering between life and death. I rolled my scooter to her side and held her hand.

With tears streaming down my face, I said, "I'll miss you very much. You've been a great friend and I love you." I glanced at her Mom and friend Dee, who sat nearby. Barb wouldn't have liked people making a fuss over her. "I know you don't want me to cry but I can't help it."

"The homeless animals of Maricopa County will miss you too, Barb. You've been their best friend. If they could speak, they'd say thank you for all you've done for them."

I wiped my tears then Barb's family, friends and I shared a group hug. I touched Barb's cheek. "I'll call Kenny now and then to make sure he's OK."

I felt the ever so slightest twitch in her hand. Even though she couldn't speak or move, she heard me. "I'm going to leave now so you can be with your family. I'll never forget you, my friend, and your great big heart."

I sobbed all the way home. Later, I cried myself to sleep. The next morning, February 22, 2002, the phone rang about 5:30 a.m. I knew it was bad news. A supervisor from the shelter called to say Barb passed overnight. I missed her more than I imagined but I was glad she was at eternal rest. She truly was the unwanted animal's best friend.

Barb wanted a memorial service but not at a church. She wasn't religious. She asked that it be held at the adoption center where she worked. On March 3, 2002, I attended my first and only memorial service at an animal shelter. The family requested an open microphone so Barb's friends and colleagues had the chance to share their experiences. Of course, I spoke about my first encounter with Barb when she looked at my scooter and asked, "Can you bring that thing to off-site adoptions?" Barb's death opened a huge gap to fill. No one hired since then ever had as much spunk as she did. The shelter was a better place for all the years she worked there. Thousands of homeless animals owed their lives to Barb Westermeyer. I owed my volunteer career at the county to her as well.

·

I wrote about my distraught feelings and pieced together a carefully worded editorial, based on my experiences at the county, and submitted it to the *East Valley Tribune* in the spring of 2005. They published it. I reworked the article and submitted it to the other daily newspaper, the *Arizona Republic*. I entered the Republic's editorial into the 2005 Cat Writer's Association annual writing contest and won a Muse Award. CWA said of my entry, "This piece stood out for actively tackling the opposing viewpoint and dismantling the arguments respectfully, piece by piece." I entered the same piece in the Dog Writer's Association of America and was nominated for an award. Obviously, there were professionals who agreed with me. Saving animals was at the forefront, but not when it came to misleading the public and to imposing unsafe or cruel conditions on the animals. I never wavered from my views.

To cope with the endless staff shortage in the kennels, the shelter tried a new approach—using inmate labor from the county jail. County inmates served short sentences, usually less than a year. I always supported giving the inmates a chance to redeem themselves. Not every man and woman incarcerated in tent city was a bad person. Most had drug and alcohol issues. Rapists, armed robbers, and murderers were locked up waiting trial but most inmates were serving time for non-violent offenses. The jail already had two animal programs running concurrently, with great success. Pleased that the shelter took advantage of men who had nothing but time on their hands, I held out hope the inmate program at the shelter would prove beneficial.

As a former social worker, the habit of trying to save human souls still lingered. I talked to the men about their convictions and tried to steer them on a path to recovery and healthy living. One thirty-something man named Ken, arrested for narcotics possession, sobbed. Ken related the story of his arrest.

"When I saw my girlfriend taken away in handcuffs, I lost it," Ken said. "I cried. I couldn't believe this was happening. I don't know how long she got."

"How long were you involved with drugs?"

"Too long."

"Was this your first arrest?"

"I've been arrested before, but it was the first for my girlfriend," Ken said. "After I get out, I've had it. No more of this life. I'm sick of it."

"Only you can change your life. There are people out there willing to help you."

"I'm planning to find them. What kind of role model are we for our kids?"

Ken was absolutely right. If he didn't want their children to follow in their footsteps, I hope he and his girlfriend dragged themselves away from the drug life.

Working with the animals soothed even the most hardened inmates. There was a surly young man named Jim. Originally jailed in Illinois for involuntary manslaughter, Jim moved to Arizona and became involved in the drug scene. He was arrested yet again. I talked to the baby-faced kid one day.

"You're so young," I said. "Is this what you want with your life?"

Jim glanced at me with puppy dog eyes. "Not really."

"If you mess up again, you're looking at serious time in Florence." Florence was a state prison where hard core criminals served time.

"Guess I got involved with the wrong crowd," Jim said. "My mom is so upset with me again."

"That's because she loves you and mothers want what's best for their children. Jail isn't what they had in mind," I said.

"I've done them wrong," Jim said. "First it was the gun thing."

Jim and his buddies bought beer and got drunk. They played Russian roulette with a gun owned by a teen's father. The boys thought the gun was unloaded. It was not. When Jim's turn came, he fired and a boy died. Jim's wealthy father paid a lawyer to help reduce the charges so Jim only served a few months in jail.

"It's not too late, Jim," I said. "Write to your family and tell them how you feel. Family can be forgiving."

"You think so?"

"Yes, but you also have to accept responsibility. When you are released, deal with your problems. Get help before it's too late."

"Guess I should," Jim said.

"We all need help now and then," I said. "Nothing wrong with that."

"I like working here around the animals," Jim said. "I feel content."

"Maybe one day you can adopt a dog or a cat."

Jim worked at the shelter for a few months. His grumpy attitude slowly melted. Around the dogs and cats, he smiled. He fed the skinny dogs extra food. When canned food was available, he doled it out to dogs and cats. He handed out treats when we had them. Every week when I came in, we always talked. I wonder if I made a difference of if Jim resorted to his old ways when he was released. I felt better for trying.

Another inmate named Santos impressed me. Like most of the others, Santos was jailed for a minor drug offense. But Santos was older than most. A Viet Nam vet, he was fifty-four years old and always called me ma'am.

"Santos, aren't you too old for this?" I said. "You served your country, fought in a war and lost your marriage because of drugs."

"Almost lost my dog too," Santos said. "My son is watching Chi Chi."

I came down hard on him because I respected him. "Is this how you want to spend the rest of your life? In jail?"

Santos gazed at the floor. "No ma'am."

"Then do something about it. Enter the drug program at the jail and stick with it once you're out," I said. "I have faith in you, Santos."

Santos worked so much harder than the others. He rarely took a break. If a dog or cat looked sad, Santos tried to rally their spirits. Every now and then, he'd say, "I'm a Marine. And Marine's do their best."

I have no idea what happened to Santos once he got into the drug rehab program at the jail. Inmates who successfully completed the program got a few weeks shaved off their sentences. I had high hopes for Santos. I wonder if he had the same for himself.

Inmates liked working at the shelter because it gave them a productive way to spend their days rather than sitting in jail learning more ways to be corrupt. For the most part, they cleaned the kennels, fed the animals, and tidied up the premises. I assumed the arrangement worked out because they always seemed busy but unfortunately problems cropped up.

At the time of the inmate program, the infamous Joe Arpaio was sheriff. He prided himself on the harsh treatment of inmates. They ate mostly bologna sandwiches. The jail sent over lunch with the inmates who worked at the shelter. Lunch, of course, was a bologna sandwich. One of the inmates looked at the sandwich and said he couldn't eat this crap. I happened to be nearby with one of the shelter dogs. The inmate offered his lunch to the dog. The dog sniffed at the food and turned his nose. I'll never forget that.

A few inmates broke the rules. Cigarette smoking wasn't allowed at the jail or at the shelter. Contraband smuggling, as I learned from various inmates, was rife at the county jail. Nicotine-addicted inmates had trouble going cold turkey. Guards on the take and visitors snuck in cigarettes, which were bartered or sold for other items like food or drugs. Guilty inmates were punished but the guard to inmate ratio wasn't large enough to keep an eye on everyone. Contraband smuggling happened at the county shelter. They couldn't figure out who was responsible but the cigarettes were always thrown out. I never caught anyone smoking or passing cigarettes but I only came in weekly.

Now and then, female workers were fearful of new inmates. I had no problems with the men but some of them looked ornery with missing front teeth, scarred faces, or grizzled skin. They obviously led tough lives but none of them ever disrespected me or the animals. After a two-year period, the shelter abandoned the inmate program. I pleaded with management to alter it rather than scrap it. Follow the procedures in place at the jail animal/inmate program. Staff interviewed inmates. Anyone with a history of violence wasn't even considered. Because the shelter program was outside of the jail, I recommended using only one or two inmates so supervision would be smoother. The shelter accepted up to five inmates and didn't interview them. Still, they were adamant and the program ended.

Most inmates were eventually released from the county jail. If they didn't receive some type of counseling or intervention, many jumped right back into the criminal life. If we wanted to end the cycle of crime, we had to help the inmates, not ignore them. The shelter program, although small in scope, had potential to intervene in their lives. Admittedly it needed to be revamped but I disagreed with shelter management. It should not have been ended. The shelter always needed the help and inmates still looked for guidance.

•

The weather was typical for summer, punishing hot temperatures and relentless sun. On my way into receiving, using the rear entry, I noticed a cardboard box that wasn't there when I left about ten minutes earlier. I stopped my scooter and peeked inside. I gasped at the sight of dead kittens. The strange car just pulling away was obviously the culprit. Inside, I told one of the employees who retrieved the box and placed them in the proper area. I felt sorry for the little ones. They never had a chance to play with yarn, try out a new scratching post, or watch birds from inside a window. At least they didn't end up as a coyote's lunch in the desert.

Other people abandoned live animals at the shelter. I caught someone in the act one morning as I cruised into the parking lot. I arrived about fifteen minutes before opening. The lot was empty except a parked car and a woman tying a dog to a pole, even though it was warm outside.

"Excuse me, what're you doing?" I asked as I drove up.

The woman stared at me. From her angry gaze, I suspected I nabbed her in the act.

"Animal abandonment is a crime in the state of Arizona," I said. "I'll serve as a witness." I took out a pen and jotted down her license plate number on a scrap of paper. Then, I got my cell phone and started to dial.

"What're you doing?" the woman asked.

"Calling the police."

"I'll wait."

"Good, the shelter opens at 9:00 a.m., fifteen minutes from now."

I drove to the employee parking lot on the side of the building. Once on my scooter, I poked my head around and checked. The woman was still there. I assumed she would wait and I went on about my business. Poor dog deserved better.

At the front desk to say goodbye to friends, Paula, the clerk, handled a transaction that I overheard. A woman turned in her dog, a handsome lab mix wagging its tail.

"Why are you turning in your dog?" Paula asked.

"Because he got too big," she said. "I got him as a puppy and I didn't think he'd get this big." This happens more than you'd think.

"What's his name?" Lucky.

I couldn't resist. "Lucky isn't too lucky, is he."

A puppy came in as a stray. That was nothing unusual. We took in stray puppies all the time, sometimes even pedigree pups. But this puppy, a sweet brown and tan chow mix with fluffy fur, had an unusual impairment. She was born without eyes. The pup sniffed her way around. She bumped into everything but she seemed healthy and happy otherwise. Because of her special needs, the Arizona Animal Welfare League, a private no-kill shelter, took her right away. They were better suited to find homes for special needs dogs and cats than we were. I hoped she went to a responsible loving home.

Animal control officers brought in a Great Dane that was seized by a local police department. The dog weighed about forty pounds, around a quarter of its normal weight. The owners claimed the dog was sick. When the ACO asked to see veterinary records the owners couldn't produce any. The owners surrendered the dog and ACOs brought him to the shelter.

"Look at this wretched dog," Stephanie, the animal control officer said, as she helped to unload the pathetic creature from the truck. "Can you believe this?"

The big brown dog, clinging to life, had an empty hollow gaze in his eyes.

"Were the owners arrested?" I asked.

"Nope," Stephanie said. She was ready to rumble. "Cops said the owners voluntarily surrendered the dog."

"That's bull," I said. "This is animal cruelty. This dog is dying from starvation. How the hell would they feel if they were starved?"

I grabbed a thick comfy blanket, filled two bowls of food and placed them in one of our larger kennels. The dog was so far gone food didn't interest him. He was sprawled across the blanket and stared at the paint chipped wall. The next day, kennel workers relieved the dog of his misery. I can't imagine the pain he endured as he wasted away.

A mother and daughter arrived with a car load full of dogs and cats to surrender. At first, I felt anger because they were parting with so many animals. As I listened further, mother and daughter were actually good Samaritans. I was too quick to judge.

"We live in a mobile home park near a mentally ill woman," the daughter said. "She's overrun with dogs and cats. Most aren't fixed either."

"She can't afford to care for them. They spent most of their days tied up outside or running loose around the park," the mother said.

"I talked to her caseworker and the park manager and we all convinced her to give them up," the daughter said. "Hope they can be saved."

"We'll do our best," David said, glancing at the dozen or so pitiful looking dogs and cats that mother and daughter unloaded from their van. All were scabby, dirty, and had mud clinging to their fur.

"They've been through a lot," the mother said. She rested her hand on David's broad shoulder. "Do your best."

About half the dogs and cats were euthanized the next day because of health and behavior problems. A few were placed for adoption. Rescue groups took the rest. The mother and daughter said they'd keep an eye out on the mentally ill woman to alert animal control authorities if she started to collect animals again.

Dogs shared the cat wing due to lack of space. Cats weren't always pleased with the constant yapping but we had no other choice. I rolled through the C wing around the noon hour to make sure the doors inside the cages were opened so the dogs had room. Workers often forgot. Others didn't care. As I rode by a cage marked "stray cat," I made a mental note to change the plaque. That was a stray white dog, not a cat.

Later on, I helped a customer interact with a cat they considered adopting. Of course I poured on all the cat's wonderful qualities. "Looking for a cat to cuddle with," the customer said.

"He'd be a great companion," I said. "Litterbox trained, knows how to use a scratching post, and he's sweet."

Out of the corner of my eye, I noticed the white dog that I thought was labeled incorrectly was actually a morbidly obese white cat. The customer left to complete the adoption and I rode to receiving to ask about the history behind the fat cat.

A worker looked up the cat's number on the computer screen. The only reason cited was moving. Immediately, I checked with Janet, the New Hope and foster care coordinator. In 2002, Janet switched jobs and joined the county. A loss for the Arizona Animal Welfare League but a huge gain for the county.

"Did you see the big girl in #336?" I asked.

"No, what about her?" Janet asked.

"It's the plumpest pussy cat I've ever seen. They must've fed her Kentucky Fried Chicken. Can you get her to a rescue group?"

"I'll do what I can. Someone should be able to help a special needs cat like this."

A woman with little dog in tow waited outside receiving. As she waited her turn in line, I noticed tears well up in her eyes. I asked what was wrong. In halting English, she said she was going to a domestic violence shelter with her five-year-old daughter. The shelter didn't accept pets. None of the area shelters accepted pets. Then her turn came. She started bawling as she handed over her dog to the clerk on duty. She begged the dog for forgiveness in Spanish, choking back tears. The bewildered dog licked her hands. I hugged the woman and said I was sorry. I promised that we would try to find a home for her dog. Once she was gone, I asked the foster care coordinator to make an extra effort to place this dog. I didn't follow-up fearing a negative response. I was truly sorry for the circumstances that led to the dog's turn in. I hope the woman and her daughter found relief at the domestic violence shelter.

I've volunteered in animal shelters since 1989, not just at Maricopa County Animal Care and Control. There's so much more to say yet there's not enough space in this book to cover all my experiences in Boston, Colorado, and elsewhere. My heart broke dozens of times by cruel, thoughtless owners who surrendered dogs and cats for trivial reasons. Watching dogs and cats try to cope from behind bars always choked me up. To them, it was like prison yet they had committed no crimes. A part of me will always cling to anger at people who gave up their old dogs and cats because it was too inconvenient to move with them. I wondered if they took their kids. You will never know the hardships you caused your pets and the people who worked in animal shelters. The abuse and neglect cases always brought tears and heartaches. I was sorry I couldn't do more to end the horrific violence in the world. All I could do was provide comfort and solace, sometimes food and soft blankets, to animals that took the brunt of human rage. It never seemed like it was enough but it was all I had to offer.

As long as there are unwanted animals, I will meet the challenge by volunteering with a rescue and/or a shelter. Only death, severe illness, or extreme disability will stop me. It's physically demanding, emotionally taxing but very rewarding.

Over the years, I met hundreds of people through animal rescue dedicated to saving the lives of abused, unwanted, and lost animals. I admired their commitment, often risking their lives, spending their own money, and working tirelessly seven days a week.

Chapter Seventeen
The Phoenix Animal Care Coalition 911

Around 2004 or 2005, I became a volunteer with the Phoenix Animal Care Coalition 911, also known as PACC911. Founder and president Bari Mears invited me to join the board. PACC911 is a multi-service non-profit that serves homeless, abused and unwanted animals in a variety of ways such as off-site adoptions, an emergency pet fund, and fundraising. During my long tenure with PACC911 (about six years) I was involved in many ways. I attended off-site adoptions and enjoyed watching pets, mostly dogs, leave for new homes. There are around 100 rescue groups affiliated with PACC911. Most are in the Phoenix area but some connect from other parts of the state. In the cool winter season, PACC911 organizes off-site adoption events at local parks, churches, car dealerships, shopping centers, or whoever invited us. The rescue groups set up adoptable animals in their assigned spaces, waiting for adopters to come along and provide forever homes. The rescue groups operated on threadbare budgets with loyal volunteers to save unwanted animals, often taken from the euthanasia list at the county animal shelter. Other times they accepted pets from abusive owners or saved them from the streets. I always admired rescue volunteers' dedication because a lot of them worked full-time jobs and had families. Rescue work occupied so much of their time. Their commitment to the cause was inspiring.

For a few years, I handled the publicity for the adoption events, sending out press releases for maximum coverage. Sometimes television stations showed up to film an animal being adopted. That was always special. There was one dog adoption in particular I'll always remember. In past years, PACC911 held an annual two-day event every October at the Franciscan Renewal Center in Paradise Valley. The church was animal friendly because St. Francis was the patron saint of animals. Throughout the long weekend, there was also a blessing of the animals. That always attracted long lines of pet owners with their beloved animals, including a lot of dogs. During a particular adoption event at St. Francis one year, the PACC911 information table was set up opposite the county adoption bus. Outside in a pen sat a lonely big brown older dog named Lady. No one adopted her all weekend. Dogs and cats that returned to the county were at risk of euthanasia. They didn't have the luxury of rescue animals that were safe in foster homes. The adoption event was slated to end at 4:00 p.m. At around 3:45, a woman adopted Lady. Everyone at the PACC911 table including me witnessed the adoption. We hugged and cried as we watched Lady's tail wag as she walked off to a better life with her new owner.

There was a tradition at PACC911 events to ring a bell every time a pet was adopted. The crowd erupted in cheers. Somehow, everyone knew what the gong signified. I still smile whenever I hear a bell ring. I think of dogs and cats leaving for good homes at PACC911 events. The bell rang particularly loud when Lady was adopted. The off-site events renewed my faith in humanity because I often met kind, caring human beings who specifically attended our events to adopt an unwanted animal. If they didn't adopt, they showed up to donate money, pet food, supplies, or offer a sympathetic word. Sometimes, they returned with a pet they previously adopted to show us how well the dog was doing. Those instances were always refreshing.

PACC911 organized an annual fundraiser called "Bowl a Rama" that lasted ten years from 2002 to 2012. I was involved for most of the ten years. The big day took months of tedious work to plan and prepare for. I attended meetings upon meetings miles from my home at a coffee shop called Coffee Bean and Tea Leaf. I didn't mind the drive because I enjoyed networking with my colleagues for a most worthy cause. I called vendors to squeeze them for donations for Bowl a Rama and other fundraisers. All money donated went toward the emergency animal fund, a source rescue groups tapped into to pay veterinary bills for injured and/or sick animals in their care. Some of the animals arrived in bad shape and needed surgery or immediate medical treatment that stretched the paltry budgets of small rescue groups. At the fundraisers we packed them in, raising thousands of dollars. I also had a heck of a good time socializing with fellow rescuers. At Bowl a Rama in particular, rescue groups dressed up in funny costumes, sang clever songs, decorated their tables, and had a relaxing afternoon away from the stress and hectic pace of animal rescue. I enjoyed every minute of it.

Chapter Eighteen
Breaking the Chain

I started Breaking the Chain in 2004 to teach third grade children about the cruelty of chaining dogs outside. I read animal magazines and learned of a woman who started an organization named Dogs Deserve Better. At the time, her name was Tammy Grimes and she devoted herself to freeing dogs tied up on chains. I ended up writing about DDB for several publications. I admired her dedication to animals and her fierce determination to end the despicable practice of chaining. Chaining bothered me too and I felt helpless to stop it. Personally, I'd never consider chaining my dogs. After reading about DDB and their expanding networks, I got the idea for Breaking the Chain. Teach children about the kindness to animals and they would hopefully influence the adults in their lives not to chain dogs.

Only two schools entered that first year, 2004. I was disappointed but not deterred. By 2005, participation tripled. By the time the contest ended in 2012, at least 4,000 children in the Phoenix area entered Breaking the Chain and benefited from a lesson on kindness to animals.

Interactive, Breaking the Chain invited children to use their creative skills to free a dog, Joey, from his chains with the help of a neighbor's cat, the Great Harriet. The goal was to teach children that animals experience pain and suffering just like they do. Although Joey is fictional, chained dogs live a miserable existence, suffering from exposure to blistering summers, frigid winters, and fierce thunderstorms. They often lack proper food and water. Chained dogs have no way to protect themselves from natural predators that inhabit certain parts of the country or from teenage miscreants who taunt and tease them. Without human touch, dogs can become vicious. Furthermore, learning about chained dogs can save a child's life. According to Dogs Deserve Better, dogs chained up to twenty-four hours a day/seven days a week kill at least fifty children every year.

Humane education, such as the Breaking the Chain contest, nurtures children's sense of empathy and kindness. Exposing them to animals in need may foster the next generation of compassionate and thoughtful leaders. Pam Gaber, president and founder of Gabriel's Angels, a pet therapy group that focuses on abused, abandoned, and at-risk children in Arizona says, "How we treat and respect animals reflects on us as a society. Breaking the Chain teaches children the importance of animals in our lives and how to treat them with respect."

The contest was sponsored by PACC911 but I raised the money, however, to award prizes to the children. We gave out prizes for first, second, and third place winners in each category, writing and art. The prizes were nominal such as a gift card to Target or Harkins theaters. Changing Hands bookstore always donated two fifteen-dollar gift cards each year for the contest. One year, I won a foundation grant to sponsor the contest. Children who won prizes were always thrilled. Sometimes their parents attended when I handed out the prizes. During the time I volunteered for Gov. Janet Napolitano, I asked for and received special proclamations for the prize winners. Students were overjoyed to receive a proclamation, signed by the governor, with their name on it. One student's art entry was so spectacular that with his mother's permission I submitted it with a magazine article I wrote about the contest. The magazine then used it for the cover. The entire family was so delighted. Each school visit was different. Sometimes I talked just to an individual class. Other times it was to the entire third grade, even if the class didn't participate in the contest. Yet there were times when the principal invited me to speak to the whole school. I felt like a super star. Me, on stage, how exciting. Children were so eager to talk about their pets. They wanted to tell me about their dogs, cats, birds, fish, horses, etc. I made sure to applaud their teachers for supporting the contest. I told them all they did excellent work even those who didn't win prizes. During our discussion, I brought up topics such as adoption, spaying and neutering, kindness to animals and to each other, as well as safety around animals. I empowered them with information about reporting animal cruelty because at least one student during every visit told a story about an animal they knew being mistreated. Children were hurt by the mistreatment of animals they cared about and they always wanted to help.

Mostly I visited the schools alone but now and then friends from the rescue community joined me to talk to the children. Candace, who then worked for a group called Maddie's Fund, brought her adopted dog Hyde. Sam who worked at the Arizona Animal Welfare League at the time came along to talk about the education programs at their shelter. Sometimes we visited schools all day, stopping for lunch at a place with a dog friendly patio of course. I treasured those days because we truly made a difference. One boy from a school in a crime-ridden section of Phoenix sent us a letter. He said that he learned a lot from our visit and that he would spend more time with his dog. That letter made all my hard work feel worthwhile. I really did make a difference.

Over the years, children produced essays and artwork that made the contest judges cry, laugh or beam with pride. There was no limit to their creativity. One boy wrote of an army of mice that chewed off the chains. "Oh my God, it's an army of mice!" screamed Joey. "No, calm down. It's just my friends. They're going to help you," Harriet said calmly. Then, the mice suddenly chewed on the chain and Joey was free.

A girl wrote of help from the police dog. "So she went to find sparking cold and icy water for the poor thirsty Joey and she did."

Another girl wrote a sad ending. "The dog died with the chain still attached to his neck. Harriet (the cat) always regretted leaving Joey (the dog) that day. Even now she could feel his pain and suffering. We shall always remember Joey now and forever."

Children always produced clever, humane, and thoughtful essays and artwork. They were a pleasure to read. More importantly, I loved visiting the schools even if I had to drive around all day, sometimes in traffic. I was sorry to see the contest end but honestly the burden for the contest fell almost entirely on me. I raised the money, I visited the schools, and I did most of the mailing to the schools. After a while I just tuckered out. I have no regrets however about all the time and effort I devoted to the contest.

·

This is the story the children read for the contest:

Harriet, a scruffy gray cat, thought she would be happy in the new house she just moved into with her owner, Candace. In the sizzling hot Arizona summers, Harriet could sit in the cool indoors and watch birds out the window all day.

After dinner that evening, Harriet jumped onto the windowsill. Instead of finding trees full of birds, she looked into the neighbor's yard and saw a big brown dog chained to a doghouse, barking loudly. Next to the doghouse sat a half-empty bowl of water. Like a wind-up toy, the dog paced back and forth. The dog's constant motion and noise made Harriet angry. She got down and looked for something else to do. Silly dog, she thought. He must be crazy.

Later the next day, Harriet heard cries from the neighbor's yard. She sped through the house to the living room for a closer look. She jumped onto the windowsill and saw the dog pawing in the dirt near the now empty water bowl. He must be thirsty, Harriet thought. She wanted to help, but how? This was a job for the Great Harriet.

A huge problem stood in her way—how to get out of the locked house. Candace, her owner, almost always closed all the windows and locked the doors before leaving for work. But sometimes she forgot to check the basement. Harriet charged downstairs and, sure enough, she found a window that was slightly open. She rammed her head against it and within seconds, she was outside.

Harriet darted across the yard and scaled the fence. She sat down by the big brown dog and asked, "What's the matter? Why are you crying?"

"Who are you?" the dog asked, too tired to lift his head off the ground.

"I'm Harriet, the greatest cat in Maricopa County. I just moved next door."

"My name is Joey and I'm hot and thirsty," the dog said, breathing heavily.

"Why are you outside tied up like a bad dog?" Harriet asked, staring at the heavy chain around Joey's neck. Her eyes followed the chain and saw that it was hammered firmly to the doghouse.

"I've been out here on this chain for three years, ever since I was a puppy," Joey said. "And I'm not a bad dog. I never bit anyone. Maybe they thought I'd run away."

"Don't get so sore," Harriet said. "What happened to your water?"

"I guess I drank it all."

"That wasn't too smart." Harriet stared at the empty bowl then looked at Joey. "Aren't you bored by yourself?"

"Sure, that's why I bark. I have no one to play with or take me for a walk."

"I just moved next door. My owner and I like a quiet neighborhood so try and keep it down," Harriet said.

"What I need is a friend. Will you be my friend?" Joey asked.

"I'm not used to having dogs as friends, but I'll think about it," Harriet said, licking her paw. "Maybe my owner can do something to get you off this hideous chain."

"I'll be your best friend if you can," Joey said as he stood up. He tried to slobber on Harriet's cheek.

"Here, here, don't get too mushy, I'm not that kind of cat," Harriet said. "But they don't call me the Great Harriet for nothing. I'll be back."

The children's assignment was to write or draw a picture providing an ending to the story. How did Harriet assist in freeing Joey? How did Joey feel once he's free? The children needed to be creative.

Chapter Nineteen
Me and the Chandler Mall

In mid-October 2001, a sprawling shopping complex including a two-level mall known as Chandler Fashion Square, opened in the East Valley area of Phoenix to rave reviews. Critics said malls were fading away and questioned whether the new mall would succeed. I shrugged off the doom and gloom. Someone always nitpicked, didn't they? To keep my mind off rumblings about an impending American invasion of Afghanistan, I drove to the new mall to see it for myself. I grew up in New York City and shopping always relieved my stress, even if I didn't buy anything. As a teenager, I visited a Rolls Royce showroom in a ritzy neighborhood wondering what it'd be like to own such an expensive car. I'm a senior citizen now and still wondering. With a skimpy budget I learned to live simply. I could squeeze a nickel until the buffalo gasped.

On that first visit to the Chandler Mall, I rode around on my motorized scooter, mostly window shopping. I passed the puppy store on the second floor and my hackles rose. As an animal lover and the owner of rescued dogs, I knew the truth behind that purebred puppy yapping in the window. I spun around, rode the elevator to the first floor and left in a huff. I refused to shell out what little money I had in a mall with a pet store. Mall pet stores procure puppies from the notoriously filthy, unsanitary, and cruel puppy mills, massive operations where female dogs are bred around their cycles. Dogs, including puppies, are treated like cheap crappy merchandise, not like the family pet. Veterinary care, regular food, and shelter from inclement weather are scarce. Puppies often arrive at the pet store riddled with disease or even dead. The Chandler puppy store was typical of all mall pet stores demanding sky high prices for purebred puppies that frequently had inbred conditions like hip dysplasia. Maybe in 2010 or 2011, I joined a feisty but dedicated group of volunteers who picketed outside local malls with pet stores including Chandler Fashion Square which, by the way, I'd stayed away from since that fall day in 2001. Because the mall was private property, we gathered on public streets holding signs saying things like "Mall pet stores buy from puppy mills" or "Adopt, don't shop." Hordes of car drivers honked in support as they pulled into mall parking lots. Now and then, someone got out of their car to inquire about our protests. We educated them about the nature of pet stores and the harsh reality of puppy mills. Due to work and school schedules, we only met on weekends for a few hours. The sizzling Phoenix summers where daytime temperatures easily spike above 110 degrees confined pickets to cooler winters.

In 2012 the unthinkable happened. The Macerich Corporation, owner of dozens of shopping malls across the nation including Chandler Fashion Square, stunned the animal rescue community. Once a pet store's lease expired it would no longer be renewed. That surprise announcement was the slow death of at least some mall pet stores. The Simon Corporation, another corporate mall owner, didn't join Macerich. Still, shelters and rescue groups were overjoyed with the decision. One by one, mall pet stores folded. More emphasis was directed toward rescued pets through dogged determination. There's a long way to go, however. Millions of dogs and cats enter shelters every year and not all of them are adopted.

The former pet store at Chandler Fashion Square became an adoption center, an extension of the Arizona Animal Welfare League, a private shelter where I've volunteered since 2008. In 2014, I moved closer to the Chandler Mall and started to volunteer there on a weekly basis.

I start my day at the mall by parking in front of Dillard's department store. Why? Just habit. Before COVID walloped us, I always arrived about an hour before my shift. I plopped myself down at the Wildflower Bread Company, a local chain of restaurants serving up good healthy food at reasonable prices, and read some of the free available newspapers, such as the *New York Times*, the *Arizona Republic*, or the *Wall Street Journal*. Wildflower featured a bread of the month and put out a plate of bread samples for customers like me to snack on. For an hour or so, I read through the newspapers and nibbled on bread slices. I then rode my scooter through Dillard's for the elevator to reach the second-floor adoption center. Breezing through Dillard's sidetracked me down memory lane. As a high school student, I worked at Macy's flagship store in Manhattan from 1970–1972. I was a waitress in a long-ago closed restaurant called the Dutch Treat. The greasy food was hardly a treat, but I was proud to earn a modest salary at the tender age of sixteen. Every late Saturday afternoon, as I walked out of Macy's, I watched fancy women in high heels and dresses at the cosmetic counter having blush, eyeliner, lipstick, etc. carefully applied by makeup saleswomen so they'd look inviting for their evening dates. My boyfriends only took me to the movies or to eat burgers and fries at cheap diners. Fond memories of my years at Macy's linger after all these years. I regret that so many chain stores buckled because of COVID and online shopping. Nothing can replace the department store. Nothing. I loved my years at Macy's.

I sign in at the mall adoption store and check out all the new arrivals. Some weeks we have a dozen puppies needing attention and a few sad-looking older dogs and cats bewildered by confinement in a cage. Maybe they wonder why their owners surrendered them. Sometimes, I wonder, too, how a ten-year-old dog or cat suddenly became a bother. To the dogs and cats (usually the older ones) I say that someone will come for you. Someone always does, even if it takes weeks. For the older dogs and cats, both staff and volunteers comfort them with cozy beds and snacks. We try to make their stay with us as pleasant as possible.

As a volunteer, I have a list of duties to keep me busy. I tackle the laundry first. Once I load a machine with soiled rags, towels, or blankets, I check to see what else needs cleaning. An empty cage is a sign that a dog or cat has been adopted. That makes me smile. I grab the disinfectant and wipe down the cage preparing the space for the next homeless pet. There's always another dog or cat ready to occupy the space. Always. Dishes, oh the dishes. The sink is filled with food bowls or toys soaking in disinfectant. I rinse them off and place them on a rack to dry. I check the clock. If it's time for the second meal, I load up a big bowl of kibble, one for puppies and one for adult dogs. Most dogs, especially the puppies, wag their tails and yip with delight when I dish out the food. Some can't wait and dig their little heads into the bowls of kibble. For those on soft food, I open up a can and scoop some into a dish.

I look into the cats' cages to make sure their food and water bowls are full. I spot check litter to make sure it doesn't need scooping. One week, I heard a desperate meow. I followed the source until I saw a cat with no food in her bowl. Maybe she was a stray and didn't get enough to eat or maybe she didn't get enough food in her prior home. I filled her bowl. That satisfied the pretty puss.

After feeding time, I'm ready to take adult dogs in the yard, a small fenced-in area outside the back entrance. There, I sit and let the dogs take care of business or wander around. Some like to play fetch. In the summer, it's smothering hot outside despite covering and sprinklers. I sometimes fill our little pool with water so the dogs can splash around. Once back inside, I sniff for poop. We don't take the puppies outside because they aren't fully inoculated yet so they eliminate in their cage. We clean up as soon as we notice waste inside. Sometimes, we place puppies in an open enclosure inside the store called the "pit." Visitors adore puppies and everyone wants to pet them. Even before COVID, we always asked people to please use hand sanitizer to prevent the spread of disease. We want to keep our animals and our customers as safe as possible.

Over the years that I volunteered at the pet adoption store, I absorbed much about mall operations. Take the loading dock for mall deliveries at the rear entry. It buzzes with activity almost all day, every day, except Sunday. UPS, FedEx, Staples, and other drivers pull up to unload goods. Employees enter and exit through the back entry as well as hang out there to smoke. Our fenced-in dog walking yard is adjacent to the loading dock but unfortunately next to a designated smoking area. Because it's outside, the rancid smoke usually doesn't bother me. Or the dogs. Once in a while, the opening and closing of truck doors scares timid dogs. So does the racket from the cardboard recycler, a huge monstrosity of a machine that crushes cardboard boxes. Employees arrive every few minutes lugging empty boxes they toss into the big machine. Once they close the door the machine emits a loud grinding noise as it compresses the cardboard. Later on, it's picked up by a recycling company to turn into more cardboard. Since we're in a locked yard, dogs can't escape. I try to comfort them, however, saying the clamor won't hurt them. Thumping music from cars waiting to pick up employees irks me, however. To me, it's not music like a soothing violin concerto but just obnoxious noise. I can't wait until the employee comes out so the driver leaves. My musical tastes are from a different era.

On the other hand, I've come to know some of the regular delivery drivers. Once a dog did get away from a volunteer. A crew of employees and volunteers mounted a valiant search for the missing dog. I asked a UPS driver with a local route to be on the lookout for our wayward woofer and he said he'd be happy to. Thankfully, a good Samaritan found the dog and returned it to our shelter. At holiday time, delivery trucks arrive non-stop. Actually, I'm glad because that's a sign of a healthy prosperous mall even if creates a ruckus.

·

COVID turned the world upside down. Few people, if any, saw the encroaching invisible enemy. The mall changed too because of COVID. In late February and early March 2020, crowds at the mall slowly thinned and nearly disappeared. Stores closed one by one. I wondered how much longer we could hold on. Soon, the governor ordered the closure of all non-essential businesses. The mall, along with our adoption store, shut down for over two months. I missed my routine of snacking on bread samples at Wildflower and reading the newspapers before my shift. I longed to hang out with the staff, volunteers, and unwanted pets.

We re-opened in mid-June to many changes. Initially, we kept the front gate down and only opened it to customers with adoption appointments. Everyone—including staff, volunteers, and customers—were required to wear masks. Only one volunteer per shift was allowed as a way to limit the number of people in the store. In the early days, the store was quiet without shoppers parading through mostly gazing at the animals. A few months later, we raised the gate and permitted a small number of people in at a time as long as they wore masks. Now we are more lenient and let in more people. More than one volunteer can work a shift but the mask mandate still stands. That's created a not so surprising pushback. Let me give you examples. Social media and the press are full of stories about the rabid anti-maskers and anti-vaxxers. Some of the dandies shop at the Chandler Mall. As a rule, an employee or a volunteer like me is at the store entrance on mask patrol. In the beginning, we charged two dollars for a disposable mask then we lowered the price to one dollar. Now we give them away for free. We ask visitors if they have a mask they can wear. Some do; some don't. Some are insulted by the question. I personally heard people say "It's just cats and dogs" to which I respond that masks protect our health. One man claimed my request was just plain stupid. He stormed away then returned to remind me how idiotic I was. I didn't take it personally. Another woman with a snarky attitude said she wouldn't come in our store if I gave her a mask. I said thank you and have a nice day. Now and then I hear people spit out curses as they pass our store that they'll never adopt from us because you have to wear a mask. Good, keep going. I wouldn't want to send one of our dogs or cats home with such belligerent people like them anyway. Another man cursed and said he'd never buy anything in our crummy store. I said to myself you probably weren't going to buy anything anyway. I am aghast at some people's hostility and level of anger.

The mall is an exciting, interesting, and mostly fun place to visit, work, shop, and to volunteer. At Christmas time, how can anyone not smile seeing children perched on Santa's lap. Each week a special adoptable dog can also sit with Santa. Why no cats? Most cats are skittish around crowds and we don't want a cat to escape inside the huge mall.

I regret that many malls face extinction from online shopping and the behemoth Amazon. How can America be America without shopping centers and malls? It's our tradition; it's in our blood. Online can never replace a day of shopping with your friends or plopping down in the food court for a sandwich or a cup of coffee. I never want to see that day happen. I hope Dillard's, Macy's, and the few remaining department stores don't meet the fate of Sears, Nordstrom's, Brooks Brothers, Century 21, and other retailers that bombed because of COVID and online competition. I'd miss the store, the volunteers, and its employees. I'd also be sad that another piece of America died and was buried. If the Chandler Mall goes, so shall our store. How can we let that happen?

Chapter Twenty
Volunteering With Refugees

Early in the summer of 2014, I moved from the trailer park, a place I had called home for the last four years. I enjoyed living in the park even though the utility bills spiked in the long, blistering hot summers, and drained my meager resources. Uninsulated, the old trailer cost a big bundle to cool in the summer. In the winter, it was cold all the time. A private charity helped pay my utility bills twice. Although I always lived on a shoe-string budget, I cobbled enough together to pay my bills with just enough left over for a movie or dinner out with friends. Having to apply for assistance was degrading. I felt defeated. I sobbed all the way to the office but felt glad that I was approved. What had my life come to, I asked myself.

There is no rent control in Arizona so the landlord raised my rent year after year. The trailer park needled me to buy the unit I rented but I declined after paying for a home inspection. With all the repairs noted, I deemed it an unworthy investment for my meager funds. I just couldn't keep up with the strangling rent increases anymore on a Social Security income so I reluctantly moved to the more conservative city of Gilbert into a barely subsidized one-bedroom apartment. I was sad to give up my little backyard where I sometimes sat outside with my dog and read a book. I relaxed on the front porch in cool weather and ate breakfast. I filled my ample storage unit with way too much stuff that I had to clear out when I moved. That was probably good because I had junk I didn't need or want. At least I didn't have to give up my dog, Franny. I cried for weeks as I packed the boxes.

I had lived in the city of Tempe for seventeen years. To me, it was home. I connected with my favorite dry cleaners, grocery stores, cafes, and knew my way around. I was a regular at the public library and the independent bookstore, Changing Hands, where I regularly attended lectures and book signings by popular authors. I lived close to the Arizona Animal Welfare League, the Sierra Club, the airport, and to a boarding kennel, all places where I volunteered. I dreaded leaving my familiar hangouts behind but, on my paltry income, I had no choice. It was the Gilbert apartment or live in my car.

The only reason I dragged myself out of bed those first few days was a warm nose nudging me. Franny wanted to eat and to go outside. Once I pushed myself off the pity pot and realized that at least I had a home, albeit one I didn't like, I slowly got back on track. I resumed volunteer work at the Arizona Animal Welfare League but at the pet adoption center at the Chandler Mall, closer to home. I was still an airport volunteer twice a week but changed to the Friday evening shift. I couldn't hack the afternoon rush hour traffic leaving at four the end of the midday shift I had previously volunteered for. I gave up volunteering for the rescue group because they moved the dogs to a Phoenix boarding kennel. I didn't feel like making the weekly drive. But I needed something else to do. Staying home in this apartment wasn't an option. I would never become an old lady, watching TV all day, or playing bingo.

The plight of refugees around the world always troubled me. The Syrian war dragged on and on with death and destruction. I no longer had cable television but the images of a nation in smoldering ruins never left me. Millions of ordinary people were displaced not just from Syria but from other nations like Afghanistan, Congo, Cuba, Somalia, Sudan, Ethiopia, and now Gaza. Aid agencies in Arizona helped them to resettle with programs like English as a second language, job placement, and computer skills. I called one of them, the International Rescue Committee (IRC), and soon became a volunteer. A global humanitarian agency with offices in the US and around the world, the IRC responds to crises such as wars, civil unrest, natural disasters, and poverty. They provide people with food, medical aid, clean water, and resettlement. At first, I wavered about making a weekly commitment because the office was in Glendale, about thirty-five miles away from Gilbert. Did I really want to drive that far every week? After my initial meeting at the IRC, a requirement for all new volunteers, I decided to give it a chance.

What changed my mind to make a nearly seventy-mile round-trip each week in sometimes crushing traffic on three different highways? The jaw-dropping presentation given at the orientation about the state of today's refugee situation convinced me that my troubles were nothing compared to the brutality faced by the refugees. My weekly drive would be a small sacrifice to help someone in need.

What if fighter jets swooped down on your neighborhood and dropped cluster bombs, flattening every building on your block? Your apartment building was badly damaged but still standing. All around you was twisted metal, toxic dust, burning buildings, and dead bodies. Your family had fifteen minutes to gather food, clothing, and vital documents then flee, hoping to find safety in an unknown place among strangers.

That's a situation that many refugees, especially the Syrians, faced. Left behind were family treasures such as photos, mementos, houses, and even pets or farm animals. Refugees also abandoned businesses that they worked years to build up. But due to the war they escaped with only the clothes on their backs. In the US, they started over, often with nothing but the meager allotment from aid agencies or handouts from charities. Refugees faced considerable challenges in their new country as they learn the language, the customs, the way of the land as well as the laws. It is not easy. The experience was humbling as well as humiliating for people, especially men, who had always been self-sufficient. I admired their strength as they worked so hard to fit in, often against neighbors who didn't believe they deserved to be here.

Once a refugee went through all appropriate background checks prior to coming to the USA, they must pass a health check, the last step in the resettlement process. If a Somali in a Kenyan refugee camp is approved for resettlement, they must travel to the capital, Nairobi, for the exam. Anyone with a communicable disease is denied entry. By the way, the vetting process is thorough and takes years. Refugees are interviewed by the US Department of Homeland Security, the United Nations High Commission on Refugees (UNHCR), the FBI, among other agencies. Refugees are fingerprinted. Interviews are thorough and lengthy. Each family member, even children depending on age, is interviewed separately. If there are discrepancies, the process is started over or ended completely. Sometimes the discrepancies are minor such as a date. A brother might say a family gathering happened in March while his sister might say April. That's minor. Wildly divergent answers, however, may indicate that someone is not being truthful. The US wants to weed out terrorists and criminals from gaining legal entry but honestly most refugees just want to escape war, civil unrest, or grinding poverty. I hardly doubt that a terrorist would submit to the rigorous vetting process that takes years or live in a squalid refugee camp waiting his turn to be resettled to a Western nation. Refugees are subject to interview after interview, questions upon questions, and even then, they may not be approved for resettlement. Memories may be shaky due to years of deprivation, lack of food, emotional trauma from living in a war zone, and the dangerous journey to relief camps. Women and girls may have been raped or sexually abused. According to the latest statistics from the UNHCR, there are around 100 million refugees worldwide and only 1% will be approved for in other countries.

Refugees are accepted by some, demonized by others, and confused at times as to where they fit in. They may hold onto old world values but their children become accustomed to American ways. Sometimes they cause conflicts at home.

Immigrant labor is vital to the American economy which would collapse without their participation. Industries such as farming, meat packing, and hospitality are dependent on immigrants to fill low-wage jobs that most Americans do not want. Crops have rotted in the fields because there aren't enough pickers. Yet there hasn't been comprehensive immigration reform in the USA since the Reagan-era of the 1980s.

Various Democratic and Republican administrations have offered reform legislation but Republican hardliners always stalled their efforts. There was no meaningful reform under the Trump administration either. So far, it hasn't happened under President Biden either.

The ESL classes I volunteered for were held four times a week for two hours a day. I volunteered just once a week. The teacher, a middle-aged man named Fadil H., asked me to come more often, but I declined due to the long distance. He understood. A former refugee himself, Fadil related to the students. He escaped from the bloody Balkan war during the 1990s, lived in a refugee camp in Macedonia then made it to the USA through UNHCR. Upon arrival, he spoke little or no English but he quickly learned because he had a wife and a family to support. He eventually became an English teacher. I bonded quickly with Fadil and enjoyed working with him. I admired his dedication to the refugees as well.

There were two levels of English classes; one for non-English speakers and one for those with some English skills. Fadil taught the class for English speakers. Another teacher taught the non-English speakers. Students in the English-speaking classes received two days of classwork, one day of conversation, and one day of computer work. I assisted in whatever way I was needed, such as making copies, one-on-one work with students, or sharpening pencils. I felt valued and needed.

All refugees who enter the USA legally come through the UNHCR. They are assigned to a resettlement agency like the IRC, Catholic Charities, or Refugees Focus who decided what city they will live in. Refugees have no say, even if they have family in the US. From the state of Arizona's Refugee Resettlement Program (paid for by the Federal Government) each family is given a small allotment of money to pay for essentials like rent, food, utilities, etc. Refugees must show they attend ESL classes, keep their medical appointments, etc. Private agencies such as the Phoenix based Welcome to America Project assist with free furniture. The State Department pays the refugees' airfare to the USA and someone from a resettlement agency meets them at the airport upon their arrival in the US. Airfare, however, must eventually be paid back. Each refugee must set up a repayment schedule with the State Department since most cannot pay back the entire sum at once. The personal allotment usually runs out in a few months so the IRC has workers available to aid refugees with job searches, teach them computer skills, and to find low-cost housing. Refugees are expected to learn English as a second language within a few months and then to find a job. Although I was only involved with the English as a second language class, I learned a lot about how the resettlement process worked from Fadil and other employees I met during my time at the agency.

Next door to our classroom was a lecture hall. Immigrants listened to an officer from the Phoenix Police Department talk about subjects such as crime prevention, emergency services, and the repercussions of criminal activity. The officer discussed the 911 system and how to summon help in case of a true emergency like a house fire or burglary. Questions were encouraged. The police also talked about local, state, and Federal laws that were applicable not just to refugees but to all Americans. The police explained that committing a serious crime like burglary or drug sales would get them deported without the possibility of returning. Traffic tickets are not deportable offenses. Most refugees are from war-torn countries so they obey all laws because they don't want to return home.

Refugees receive work permits so they can legally seek employment. They can also attend school or job training programs. After a few years, they can apply for green cards, which enables them to become permanent residents. The next and last step is citizenship. The entire process from entry as a refugee to citizenship takes about ten years. Children born here, of course, are automatically citizens.

Once in the US, refugees are given appointments with the county health department for yet another exam as well as vaccinations which includes a tetanus shot. These appointments must be kept. If one is missed for whatever reason, it must be rescheduled. A refugee must bring proof to the IRC that he received the appropriate medical exam and vaccinations.

Class sizes in the ESL varied. One week there might be a full room with as many as twenty students. The following week, there might only be ten students. Why the difference? Refugees had various appointments to keep, set up by the IRC. There were appointments with the health department, Social Security, to enroll children in school, job interviews, etc. They sometimes missed a bus connection. Few, if any of the refugees, owed a car. Some had friends who gave them a lift. Phoenix has one train system that isn't close to the IRC. The region is served by buses but they are not always reliable. If a connection is missed, the wait for the next bus might be half an hour. Students also dropped out when they found jobs. Some moved to other cities where they had friends or families. I always celebrated when someone obtained employment or moved in with relatives. Their success reinforced my commitment to the program.

Students came from a variety of backgrounds as well as ages. Some were young, maybe 19 or twenty years old while others were old enough to be grandparents. Most refugees to Arizona were from Afghanistan, Somalia, Iraq, Congo, Cuba, Ethiopia, and Mexico. There were doctors, lawyers, teachers, and architects, as well as common laborers. Some were Christian while others were Muslim, Buddhist, or Hindu. Anyone with an advanced degree was at disadvantage because of strict American retraining rules and requirements. A doctor from Syria, for example, would have to complete a three-year residency in his field to practice medicine in the USA. Before seeking a residency for which they were paid, refugees had to be skilled in English. Architects, nurses, engineers, lawyers, and others had to complete similar retraining, which could be costly as well as time consuming. Many refugees had families to support and didn't have the time or money for the required classes so they worked in their fields but in lesser positions. Nurses, for example, may work as nurse's assistants or as X-ray technicians. Lawyers might work as paralegals. But the refugees seemed satisfied with gainful employment in a nation at peace. Other refugees took menial jobs as housekeepers, maintenance workers or fast-food cooks. At the same time, they enrolled in community college classes to improve their skills for better paying jobs.

Students from each nationality grouped themselves together. For instance, Cubans sat with Cubans, Somalis sat with Somalis, and Congolese sat with Congolese. To encourage friendships, Fadil broke up the students and made them sit next to someone they didn't know. Some hedged about moving but eventually they grew comfortable sitting next to someone from another country. In fact, a young woman from Somalia—who I'll call Fazia—became so friendly with a Mexican lady named Maria that she once chased an Afghan man who sat next to her. Fazia arrived a little later than usual and the Afghan man took an empty seat available which happened to be next to Maria. Fazia stood in front of him said I'm sorry sir but I always sit next to Maria, you'll have to sit somewhere else. Fadil and I looked at each other and smiled.

A few months later, I once met a young man, a maintenance worker, at the airport where I volunteer. He looked familiar and we greeted each other. From the Congo, he was in the English class at the IRC where I assisted. I honestly didn't remember him but he was now a supervisor in the airport maintenance department. I said how proud I was of him and wished him well.

There was an immigrant, a young man from Iraq, who lost part of his left arm in a bomb blast back home. Finding a job was a challenge because of his disability. His intellect, however, was sharp. I sometimes chatted with a guy at the gym, Max, where I exercise. Max was born with part of his right arm missing. His parents raised him to be like every other kid in the neighborhood. I asked Max what advice I could give the young man from Iraq about finding a job.

"Look for a job at a call center," Max said. "That doesn't require two hands. Workers at those jobs use headsets. If they use a computer, no problem. I use a computer with one hand. This guy probably already does too."

"Good idea," I said. "I'll let him know."

"Tell him not to give up either," Max said.

On my return the next week, I passed along Max's advice. I hope it helped. About two weeks later, I no longer saw the Iraqi. Perhaps he found a job. He was an intelligent, kind young man eager to work.

Nearly all the immigrants I met were eager to work, learn English or to attend college.

Refugees with children in the public-school system are at a distinct advantage. The public schools employ ESL teachers who immerse foreign students in English so they become proficient much quicker. Children of refugees help their parents pick up the language at home. Until they are secure in their language abilities, we encourage the refugees to speak only English at home. We didn't want them to lose their cultural heritage but until they are comfortable with English, speaking it at home was for their own benefit. We suggested reading English newspapers for magazines out loud, borrowing CDs or DVDs from the public library or watching television. Other refugees from prior classes reported that aided them as they studied English.

Some refugees found jobs right away. Not feeling totally confident with their English skills, they returned to ESL classes for improvement. I heard from several refugees that fellow employees helped them with English while on the job. Now and then, a refugee talked of family members, already in the US, who worked with them on English skills. All the extra assistance was beneficial.

I learned a lot from my interactions with the class. Some refugees were almost illiterate in their native language, whether it was Spanish, Arabic, Hindi, or whatever. I don't know what they did in their native countries. Maybe the women didn't work, maybe they did. I don't know. Picking up English was difficult on some no matter how hard they tried or how much individual attention me or Fadil provided. I wondered how they would find a job because time was of the essence. Refugee programs only carry them along for a few months. After that, they are on their own. Others arrive with families that include 10 or 11 children. By American standards, that's a large family. If the parents worked menial jobs skills back home, which was frequently the case, I wondered how they secured jobs in Arizona that paid enough to provide for such large families. Rent in Phoenix is less expensive than in cities like San Francisco, New York, and Chicago, but still it is not cheap. Refugees can apply for public housing and/or Section 8 but those government subsidized programs are in high demand and short supply. I always hoped they succeeded having come from so far away with dreams and aspirations. Once in a while, I heard of refugees who gave up and went home. Making it in America was too hard on them. Life can be challenging for Americans too.

There is also the issue of emotional trauma. A lot of refugees arrived with the nightmares from war, civil unrest, drought, rape, or living in overcrowded camps. One woman said she had to wrap her children in plastic at night to keep the scorpions from biting them. Children, especially the Syrians, may not have been to school for months or even years or they attended sporadically. The children may now have trouble adjusting in the rigors of daily school and all its requirements. Parents may be unprepared to hold any kind of job. The greater Phoenix community, Christians, Muslims, and Jews, collectively work together to see that refugees succeed. I am in awe of the volunteers and paid employees who work tirelessly on behalf of the refugees. Their dedication and zeal is inspirational as well as uplifting. Without their support, caring and concern, Arizona's refugees could not have resettled without them.

A few refugees came from countries that experienced weather related trauma such as earthquakes or hurricanes. There were a few students from Nepal and Haiti, countries that were barely hanging on and then they were struck by disastrous earthquakes. Not only was Haiti ravaged by a major earthquake in 2010 that killed thousands and wrecked the country, but Hurricane Matthew blasted the island in 2016. That storm dumped torrential rain, leaving thousands homeless and killed hundreds. In the two and a half years I was at the IRC, I only recall one student who was from Haiti. I met a few now and then from Nepal.

Once a week, Fadil chose a student to talk about his homeland and his journey to the USA. A middle-aged Muslim man from Iraq, Faisal, talked about the vagaries of life in the Saddam Hussein years. Ruthless and cruel, Hussein kept strict order and control. According to Faisal, people generally got along. Faisal had Christian neighbors. No one bothered with the Yazidis. Life could be rough but Faisal went about his business. On weekends, he played cards with his friends. He had a job, a family, and a home. Then the US invaded in 2003, Hussein was killed, and the country disintegrated into madness. Fighting broke out and escalated across the country, enveloping neighbor against neighbor. When the militants known as ISIS came, Faisal said it was time to leave. He wanted no part of them or the grisly version of Islam they spread. He considered himself one of the lucky ones to resettle in the US. So many others were left behind. He misses the old Iraq when there was peace, even if it meant having a dictator Hussein in rigid control. At least people weren't killing each other. Hussein killed his opponents but more or less left the citizens alone as long as they didn't complain about his rule.

Fadil related to Faisal's story. He lived in the former Yugoslavia in what he calls a benign communist nation. The dictator, Marshal Tito ruled from 1953 until he died in 1980. After that, the nation of Serbs, Croats, and Bosnians, that once lived as neighbors, slowly broke apart into a punishing civil war that lasted from 1992 until 1995. Europe had not witnessed war since the 1940s. Thousands died, were injured, or displaced. A nation that once hosted the Winter Olympics in Sarajevo in 1986 was in ruins. Yugoslavia later splintered into six different countries after the Dayton Peace Accords in 1995. Even with the presence of UN Peacekeepers, it is still hard to keep a lid on age old hostilities.

From the Cubans, I learned how the decades old economic embargo failed miserably to bring down the dictator Fidel Castro or to end the communist regime. Castro died on November 25, 2018, and the island still clings to communism. The former communist USSR was Cuba's benefactor that sent oil, food, machinery, spare parts, etc. in exchange for sugar and citrus but when the government broke apartment in the early 1990s, Cuba lost its largest and most important trading partner. Strongman Hugo Chavez rose to the dictatorship of Venezuela in 1999. He, too, supplied Cuba with vital supplies such as oil and food but the island was again sent adrift when Chavez died in 2013.

Castro and Communism have outlasted the embargo which only brought misery and deprivation to the island and her peoples. Even though citizens are given food coupons each month, they are essentially worthless because grocery stores face persistent lack of essential items like fresh meat, rice, salt, eggs, cereals, fruits, vegetables, etc. A thriving black market exists as a result. Those with money buy needed goods but at higher prices. The poor just do without. The average Cuban worker earns about ten dollars a month. Doctors and other professionals make a little more, maybe forty dollars a month. It's nearly impossible to live a decent life unless a Cuban has family and/or friends outside the country who send regular remittances. The embargo has brought pain and suffering to Cuba but communism has failed them miserably too.

Buildings, both residential and commercial, are in disrepair. Buses are old and decrepit, coughing out toxic fumes as they carry around passengers to work or to visit family and friends. Medical care is free as is education but there are shortages of essential supplies. Most Cubans do not own cars. Spare parts are hard to find.

A Cuban student once said, "We go anywhere. To any country that'll have us."

Many Cubans flock to Spanish speaking countries because of the language. A student said Ecuador and Spain were common destinations. But many Cubans eventually find their way to the USA because other nations often do not offer permanent residency or a path to citizenship. They may acquire a long residency or a work permit but no other guarantees. In the USA, on the other hand, a refugee can work toward citizenship, if no serious crimes are committed.

Prior to resettling in the US, a young Cuban man said he lived for a while in Ecuador working as a waiter. Single and childless, he could only afford to send twenty-five dollars home each month to his family. That amount, however, can be stretched to buy food or clothing for a few months. Another Cuban refugee said that if someone doesn't have a relative or friend to send remittances, neighbors with the extra help share their food and supplies. Deprivation made the Cubans resourceful as well as caring.

One student described a typical weekend activity. A group of friends and neighbors would pack a picnic lunch. Few people owned a car so they piled onto the local bus and rode to the beach. They drank a few beers, sodas, and passed around sandwiches. For entertainment, someone brought along a radio. They listened to music and danced. The refugee said it was one of the only forms of relaxation—a picnic at the beach. They couldn't afford anything else. Movie theaters, plays, or dinner out just wasn't possible for the average Cuban.

Not every Cuban was happy to be in the US. I noticed a middle-aged Cuban woman crying in class once during an individual assignment lesson. I asked her what was wrong.

"I miss my country," Lourdes said. "I didn't want to leave."

"Sorry that you're sad," I said.

"I don't like it here, but I can't live on $10 a month in Cuba. So hard for me and my son."

"I bet it is," I said. "Do you have friends or family here?"

"Not in Phoenix, but in Miami."

"Maybe you can move there."

"That's my plan. My family is saving up for my plane ticket," Lourdes said. "I am too. I got a job recently."

Every week, when a refugee talked about his country of origin, my own horizons expanded. A Congolese man, older and mature, always wore a suit and tie to class. He looked so dapper and sharp. He talked once about food back home. It all sounded delicious until the delicacy made from snake. A teacher, a young man from Rwanda, worked hard to hone his English skills to secure a position as a teacher here in the US. He thought American teachers didn't receive the same level of respect as they did in Rwanda. The idea that a parent would sue the school because a student failed a class was unheard of in Rwanda. Students arrived in class on time, dressed properly, didn't listen to cell phones, and spoke with courtesy to teachers. There was no gun violence either. Wow, imagine that in the USA.

A sweet refugee, a young man from Afghanistan, had married just before he received the go ahead to immigrate to the USA. Big fancy weddings were popular in Afghanistan. Lots of people from both sides of the family were invited as well as friends, co-workers, neighbors, and friends of friends. The invitation list can be very long. The Afghan student said saying no to someone who wants to attend your wedding is an insult. No family wants to be known as the one who turned their back to a wedding guest. A wedding hall rental plus the food can cost a bundle but it was tradition. The refugee said it cost him and his family a huge amount of money but he seemed happy. A Nepalese man talked of the hardships of life in a refugee camp in Thailand where he lived for several years before the UNHCR approved his request to emigrate with his wife to the USA. He seemed most thankful to live here. Once he was settled and found a job, he planned to do volunteer work in some capacity as a way to say thank you.

After two and a half years, I left the IRC. The long weekly drive grated on my nerves. Fadil and I kept in touch for a while but we eventually stopped calling each other. He'll always remain dear to me. The experience with refugees was inspirational, touching as well as educational. Even though I personally live in subsidized housing and have applied for outside assistance for food and utility bills several times in recent years, I have not endured war, civil unrest, or a devastating natural disaster. I am blessed compared to the harsh experiences shared by some of the refugees I had the pleasure to work with. They truly made my life better. I hope I did the same for them.

Chapter Twenty-One
My Journey to Islam

That unforgettable day in September 2001 shifted my attention to Islam. For years, religion played little or no role in my life, even though I was raised Catholic and attended Catholic schools. Indeed, I started to shun religion as a child. I was turned off by the way Black people were treated during our visits to my mother's family in rural Alabama at the edge of the Jim Crow era. In school, the nuns taught us that God loved everyone. From what I observed, it didn't seem that God loved Black people. There was a small grocery store in our Queens neighborhood where I bought my father's cigarettes. An older man worked there named Ziggy. Balding with a sad face, I noticed faded numbers tattooed onto his hairy arms. I asked him about the numbers one day. He said I wouldn't understand. Some months later, I asked him again about the numbers. Ziggy said he was in a death camp during World War II. A lump clogged my little throat. Who would hurt lovable Ziggy? Although quiet, he was always nice to us children, often treating us to candy. I felt awful. What was a death camp anyway? I'd never heard of such a terrible thing so I asked my parents but they couldn't quite explain the evils of the Holocaust. Neither did my Catholic school teachers, all nuns. I wondered why God didn't seem to love the Jews, although I didn't know any Jews except for our family doctor. What harm could they have done to deserve the death camp? I grew up in a segregated all white ghetto. If a Black family even so much as ventured through the community, the neighbors shrieked with disgust as well as fear. What will happen to our neighborhood if the "colored" move in?

Well, as it happened, a Cuban family did move in. I don't remember much about them except they played cards and had a big black dog aptly named Blackie. I always loved animals but we never had pets in our family. My mother always said no. I asked the Cuban family if I could visit and play with Blackie. They said yes but of course my mother said no, I couldn't enter the Cuban's apartment. My father always deferred to her. The Cuban family let me play with their dog but only in the hallway. I don't know what perceived harm my mother thought the Cubans might do to me in their apartment. She did, however, permit me to visit the Greek family who lived on the same floor. I was confused and uncertain about race. Why could I visit the Greeks but not the Cubans? She couldn't explain it either yet I was expected to understand. My dad always read the newspaper each morning before he left for work. As I ate breakfast, I read the paper out of boredom as it sat there on the kitchen table. I remember reading about the US military dropping napalm bombs on Vietnamese children, children like me, in the 1960s. The stark photos of frightened children running away, sometimes naked, from American caused explosions sickened me. Why were we doing that to children in far-away lands who seemed like no threat to the USA? After high school graduation, I lost interest in religion and attending Sunday mass, a requirement for Catholics. Undoubtedly, I disappointed my mother who was a devout Catholic but the church meant little to me.

I always believed in God, however. Throughout life I attended Christian services now and then but mostly out of fear that if I didn't show up God would punish me. Honestly, though, I had no interest otherwise in Christianity but the fear of the devil that my mother instilled in me as a child lingered well into adulthood.

After the car accident of 1994, I believe God spared me for a reason. I could have easily died that day but I didn't. Plenty of people perish or are seriously impaired in car accidents every year, especially in pedestrian car accidents like mine. I survived and decided to find out why. Over the next decade, I church shopped but nothing fit. I went mostly to satisfy my debt to God for sparing my life. I even tried a Buddhist temple and a Quaker service. Still nothing worked so I moved onto spiritual services at the Southwest Center for Healing Arts in Tempe, a new age school that teaches yoga, meditation, reflexology, etc. I attended healing ceremonies on occasion and felt reasonably satisfied. I also attended monthly laugh groups where we laughed for no reason. Yes, we just laughed. Yet something was lacking in my life. I couldn't plug up the empty feelings. My soul wasn't fulfilled. I needed something more. What?

The media madness swirling around Islam after 9/11 poisoned our perceptions about people and a religion I didn't know much about. Why condemn over a billion Muslims for the horrific actions of a few? After watching the news coverage of the Twin Towers, I took out the Yellow Pages (yes, phone books existed back then!) and I called all the mosques in the Phoenix area. For anyone who picked up the phone, I said I hoped that there wouldn't be a backlash against Muslims. I offered prayers for peace and harmony. That would surely be needed in the days ahead. I followed the news with even more intensity as the Bush administration prepared for inevitable war in the Middle East. The world would never again be the same.

Once the hysteria of 9/11 died down, I started riding my motorized scooter near the Tempe Mosque, wondering what it was like inside. I'd never been inside a mosque before. Now and then I'd see men or women outside but I was too timid to approach anyone. What would I say? I supposed I could have just said something simple like hello. I continued down the street, usually stopping at the now defunct Border's Books and Music on Mill Avenue to browse around the bookshelves and to drink coffee. A local newspaper article one day grabbed my attention. I don't remember the year. Vandals scrawled ugly, vulgar graffiti on the Tempe Mosque, making me feel sad. It must've been a Friday, the Muslim holy day, because there were dozens of people milling about outside as I rode past. Sucking up my fears, I proceeded to a group of women. I apologized for the crude and insensitive actions of the vandals who defaced the mosque. Although religion meant little to me at the time, I recognized its importance to others. I would have denounced the vandals had they struck a church, temple, or other place of worship. The Muslim women accepted my good wishes and suggested I return for a Friday prayer service. I was dressed in a T-shirt, jeans, and sneakers, not appropriate attire for the mosque. I said I would return but never did.

Borders Books and Music eventually closed after the chain filed for bankruptcy so my downtown hangout was gone. On occasion, I watched activity at the mosque if I ate at the Middle Eastern café next door with friends, always curious but never brave enough to make a move and attend a service. There were logistical concerns. What would I look like in a hijab? Without proper supervision, my head scarf would probably be lopsided and dorky. If the weather was windy, the scarf would probably sail off my head. Buried underground my interests lay dormant but resurfaced years later.

Finally, in September 2011, I went through my morning ritual, sipping coffee and reading the newspaper when I noticed an advertisement for an interfaith service at the Tempe Mosque to commemorate the ten-year anniversary of the 9/11 attacks. Hailed as a celebration of peace and understanding, Christians, Jews, Muslims, and anyone else interested was invited to attend the event. A friend joined me. The imam ordered chairs for 30 people. Over 300 people attended. It was an awesome evening of friendship, caring, and spirit of diverse people devoted to a better world. On the way out, Muslim volunteers handed out Qurans. I took one home and placed it on my bookshelf. I never read it. I never read the Bible either.

My interest in Islam lingered although I told no one. As the internet picked up speed, I checked out websites and Facebook pages on Middle East animal rescue. There were at least a dozen groups perhaps more in Saudi Arabia, Egypt, Iran, Kuwait, Turkey, Lebanon, and beyond. Slowly, I started to make connections and chatted with people online. Eventually, I met a middle-aged woman, Maha, from Saudi Arabia. Although we've never met in person (I hope we do), we've been friends online for about five years. A devout Muslim, she once asked about my Quran. I meant no disrespect to Islam but the Quran was still snuggled safely on my bookshelf.

"Why don't you read it?" Maha suggested. Why don't I? I started to read the Holy Book, taking a year to eventually finish. During that time, Maha and I engaged in many discussions about Islam. She also sent me other books about Islam from Saudi Arabia, which I've read through as well. I then read a book called the *First Muslim*, an intriguing book about the life of Muhammad. My interest grew steadily. I still did not, however, return to the Tempe Mosque for Friday prayers.

Everything changed when I started as a volunteer at Sky Harbor airport in the fall of 2010. At the airport, Muslims came into my life. I met numerous Muslim employees working as housekeepers, baristas in Starbucks, clerks in retails stores, driving intra-terminal buses, taxis, limos, baggage handlers, and more. I became friendly with several Somali women, especially one named Qamar. Every time we saw each other we talked. Then in the spring of 2013, Qamar broke the delightful news about her first pregnancy. She'd be leaving soon for maternity leave. As a gesture of good will, I brought a gift for the baby. About four to five months later, she sent me an email along with a baby picture with a suggestion to visit. At the time, we lived only about ten minutes apart so I visited Qamar and her infant daughter Salmo often. Ever since then, we've become good friends. Salmo is like the granddaughter I never had. Qamar her husband Said are kind, caring, and loving people devoted to their children and their faith. I am blessed to have them in my life. I was honored to attend Qamar's swearing in ceremony when she became a US citizen in 2014. From them, I learned more about Islam.

Around the spring of 2013, I met Nadia, a Pakistani American at the airport. At the time, I was stationed at a post behind security. She had asked me for a place to pray. Ordinarily, I would have suggested the interfaith chapel but it was outside of security. I pointed out a quiet corner nearby. We chatted for a bit then exchanged contact information. A skilled artist with international connections, Nadia is also a devout Muslim who further piqued my interest in Islam. She says her artwork is inspired by Islam. About six months later, Nadia contacted me. She was on a business trip with a connection in Phoenix. I met her for lunch. What a delight to see her again.

And then I met Diba, who has become my dearest friend and my sister. A simple smile brought surprising changes into my life in July 2013 when a middle-aged Muslim woman wearing a colorful hijab stood outside a security checkpoint.

"Do you need help?" I asked.

"No, thank you," she said, watching passengers enter and leave the secured area. "I'm dropping off family. They're flying back to Virginia"

"OK," I said. "I hope they have a safe journey home."

Our casual encounter continued. Warm feelings lingered. I didn't want to leave and neither did Diba. Away went her cell phone and we both started a new phase in our lives. I explained my motorized scooter and Diba, too, was seriously injured in a car accident. Throughout my now almost eight-year tenure at the airport, I've had intimate conversations with passengers about their lives. I couldn't let Diba leave without asking if we could get together. Of course, she said, handing me a slip of paper with her phone number. Ramadan, the most sacred Muslim holiday, approached so Diba said we'd meet afterwards. She'd be fasting all day for four weeks, a tradition followed by all able-bodied adult Muslims during Ramadan. I understood and looked forward to sharing a meal with her soon.

After that first meal, Diba and her family embraced me as one of their own. Not only have I shared meals with Diba and her husband, Abdul, but I was invited to numerous family gatherings. From sharing food and conversation, I've learned so much about Afghan culture.

Afghan people are thoughtful, generous hosts. As soon as I enter an Afghan home, there are always plates of food, sweets, and green tea. Drinking green tea is an Afghan tradition.

On a lazy Saturday afternoon in the fall of 2013, I stopped at an ATM after leaving the gym. A surprise call from Diba invited me to join her at the hospital to visit her sister-in-law Maniga who had surgery. "Sure," I said, "I'll meet you there." Inside a small hospital room, at least a dozen Muslim women surrounded Maniga with well wishes. We all talked and laughed. On my way out, I saw more women in hijabs carrying flowers and gifts on the way to see Maniga. I was impressed by the outpouring of support and concern from the Afghan community for their sister Maniga.

I once joined Diba for an Islamic memorial service. The loosely fitting scarf was a bit to one side on my head, not quite covering my hair like other Muslim women but I looked presentable. I learned more and more about Afghan customs and traditions. To add to my growing knowledge, I took out books from the library. I read about the misery created by the Soviet invasion, the ensuing violence, and the cruelty imposed by the Taliban. I gobbled up information as fast as I could. On the Friday before she moved to California, I attended my first Friday prayer service at the Chandler Mosque.

Diba and Abdul moved to southern California in late November 2013 to be closer to their only daughter, where she attended graduate school. Seeing the moving truck pull away that Saturday afternoon nearly broke my heart but I understood. I missed Diba so much but we're in contact almost every day. Her family considers me one of their own so I see them as much as I can. I wish visits were more often but they have busy lives and families.

During Ramadan 2014, I joined Diba's family and friends for evening Iftar's (breaking the fast) at an Islamic center in Chandler. I cherished my evenings sharing home-cooked food, conversation, and prayers with my sisters, some of whom I met for the first time. Women laughed, hugged, and traded bits of our lives as we sat around and enjoyed home-cooked food. Children played under watchful adult eyes. After eating, we took turns cleaning up. And then at the end of July, Ramadan was over. There would be no more evenings at the Islamic center. I didn't want it to end. I loved the camaraderie among Muslim women. No one was a stranger. Everyone including me was welcomed. I missed my sisters. I hope they missed me too.

In the summer of 2013, as I soul searched Islam, I discovered AMWA (American Muslim Women's Association of Arizona). I read of their toy drive during Ramadan. For seven years I was a pet therapist with Gabriel's Angels, an all-volunteer group that tries to break the cycle of violence in abused, abandoned, neglected, and at-risk children through healing pet therapy. My adopted dog Luke and I visited a homeless shelter. At Christmas time, friends donated gifs for the children. Those small presents boosted their spirits. I imagined that Ramadan gifts would be just as uplifting for Muslim children so I donated a few toys. AMWA's Facebook page listed several drop off locations, one of which was the Tempe Mosque. When I left the toys, no one was there. Just the box. I had wanted to meet the women involved so I noted their annual meeting on my calendar and showed up, scared, and alone. Diba joined me there. I continued my affiliation with AMWA, however, growing more comfortable each time I attended an event. I respected AMWA's commitment to women in the community and their devotion to improving lives of new refugees. I served on the board of AMWA during 2015.

And lastly there was the MSA (Muslim Student Association) at Arizona State University. I wish I could start over again so I could hang around with these energetic, enthusiastic, and motivated young people. That's an impossible dream so I admire and support them, wish them well and hope they can change the world in a way our generation failed to do. I'm from the Woodstock era. It's not that we didn't try but along the way so much has happened. The world today is twisted by war, hatred, poverty, and extremism that threaten our very existence.

I attended an interfaith dinner sponsored by the MSA in 2014 and again in 2016. What awesome evenings. I made new friends in 2014, Sarah and Mohammad, who have become like family to me. I was sorry when they moved back to Saudi Arabia in 2015 after completing their studies in the USA. Over the years, I enjoyed the company with lots of ASU students at Islamic Awareness Week, Friday prayer services and other community events. What more could I ask for?

I started attending Friday prayer services weekly in late summer of 2014 and haven't missed once since. Imams or guest speakers only talk of love, kindness, caring, and family. There is no talk of hatred. Ever. At family gatherings, there is always food, fun, and lots of sharing. At community events, people join for the common good such as raising money for hunger or to help refugees settle in. No one had to ask me to become Muslim. Their behavior showed me the true meaning of Islam. Don't be fooled by the few who strayed and shame us all by their frightful behavior. I've experienced nothing but love, compassion, and caring. I hope it never ends either.

Along my journey, there were some interesting experiences before I said the *shahada* or the declaration of faith to Islam. Take the time I participated in World Hijab Day that takes place every February 1. How would my friends react to me in a hijab, the Muslim woman's head covering? The first World Hijab Day was intended to bring understanding and friendship among Muslims and non-Muslims.

Started by New Yorker Nazma Kahn in 2013, non-Muslim women and uncovered Muslim women were encouraged to wear a hijab for a day. Spread largely through social media, the event drew thousands of supporters from around the world. I participated too although I'd worn a hijab before at an Islamic memorial service and the first time I went to a mosque with Diba. Respecting tradition I wore a hijab when it was expected. I hedged at first about wearing a hijab on February 1, 2014 without the company of Muslim friends in my comfort zone. What would people think? Then I said who cares what people think or say. It's my head. I'll cover it if I choose. I showered, changed, then draped a pretty blue scarf around my gray hair. I met my friend Julie for breakfast at a local café. My appearance was uneventful to nearly everyone except for a man sitting nearby. He glared at me throughout our casual breakfast of pancakes and coffee. He must admire a gorgeous older woman with her head covered.

Feeling more confident in my hijab, I drove to a pet adoption event where I was expected as a volunteer. Only one head swerved. Her eyes rolled too. I said I'm proud to spread kindness friendship and harmony in the world. To the rest of my friends and colleagues, I was the same person I always am—friendly, a bit nutty, and congenial. The homeless dogs and cats of course could care less what I wore. They never do. After the event, I went food shopping. No one paid attention to an older disabled woman squeezing melons in the produce section or riding around in her scooter with a basket full of fruit and Brown

Cow yogurt. At the end of the day, I felt proud for leaving my comfort zone. Muslim women are not alone in covering their heads. Catholic nuns, Orthodox Jews, Sikhs, and Hindus all wear head coverings. Even the ex-slave Harriet Tubman is pictured with a head covering. World Hijab Day was a step to overcome prejudice and fear of Islam. If there is a second annual World Hijab Day, I'll take part. Little did I realize I was well on my way to becoming a Muslim.

Islam formally came into my life in February 2015 when I said *shahada*, or the proclamation of faith that was a formal conversion to Islam, after years of introspection, reading, talking, searching the internet, and attending Friday prayer services. I said it first with my friend Saba, after a Quran group meeting at ASU. A few days later, how many, I'm not sure, but I was at the Friday prayer services at the Tempe Mosque when I heard an announcement that a sister was saying the *shahada*. It was me! After I repeated the declaration, all the sisters warmly welcomed me with hugs and well wishes. I received several gifts too during the following weeks. What changed since then? Everything and nothing. I still enjoy a gut busting joke, remain devoted to my friends, and never touch junk food. Ever. I'll die loving animals and protecting the environment. Nothing can shake my devotion to peace and prosperity in the world. Books and the printed word hold me as they always have. I enjoy seeing a good movie. Drinking coffee and reading an interesting book at a local café makes my day. I love to share a tasty meal with friends. A lively game of Scrabble is a favorite.

Converting to Islam, however, changed so much. First, it brightened my social life and ended years of boredom and loneliness. There are always happenings at local mosques, such as group activities, lectures by guest speakers, or fundraising dinners for worthy causes. On Super Bowl Sunday 2015 a new friend invited me to watch the big game with her family and friends. My preferred team lost but who cares. We've had lunch after Friday prayer services and breakfast on Sundays. I am invited to potluck dinners. Another sister who lives nearby asked me to visit and we started to play Scrabble. I developed another friendship with a sister and her three sons. We eat lunch often, take her boys to a play area at a mall, and sometimes go for a ride outside the city. A group of sisters once in a while enjoys coffee and conversation at Starbucks or socializes in a public park. I've made friends with sisters visiting from outside the USA and learning about their culture. My Somali friend cooks for me often and I love playing with her children. I became close friends with a sister and her son from Saudi Arabia. They are like family too. Now and then, a local mosque organizes a family picnic in a park and everyone shows up for food, friendship, and faith. The invitations continue weekly. Sometimes I say no because they interfere with my regularly scheduled volunteer work. I am humbled by the warmth, love, and care my sisters and their families have shown me.

Love is like the wind, you don't see it but you feel it. That's an apt way to describe the sisters in my halaqa, also known as a Quran study group that I began to attend in the early part of 2015. Starting out with a potluck dinner, we nibble on homemade food and dabble in conversation about our lives, families, jobs, friends, or the latest news. Then it's time for business. A smart, well-read sister leads us in discussion on parts of the Quran. We ask questions and talk about true Islam, not the distorted often violent version a few misguided and fanatical men carry out in the name of Islam. At either Maghrib or Isha, depending on the time of year, we break to pray together then return to finish our discussion. We end with a sister (which now is often me) offering up a prayer of peace, mercy, or thanks. Our Quran group is diverse with women ranging in age from students to seniors. Women come from around the world including places like Somalia, Egypt, Morocco, Algeria, Chile, Puerto Rico, Afghanistan, Tunisia, Ethiopia, Pakistan, Malaysia, Bangladesh, Mexico, and the US. Forgive me if I left out someone's country. Our differences enrich us yet we are bonded by our devotion to Islam and to each other. For a long time, I knew little or nothing about Islam but the more I learn, the more I want. My sisters help me expand my knowledge. It's refreshing to be in a group without competition, gossip, or backbiting. We respect each other and truly care about one other's well-being. There's no rivalry on who has the sharpest looking purse or most expensive hijab. We're in this together as sisters in Islam. If I fail or if I succeed, at least I know my sisters are on my side. This is the true face of Islam. Thanks, ladies, for welcoming me into the group. I am truly blessed.

Every religion has standards; Islam is no different. Women and men are encouraged to be modest. I cover my head with a hijab, wear long sleeves blouses and skirts, as well as knee-length tunics. I bought my first abaya last July during Ramadan 2015. The sister selling abayas and hijabs outside the mosque suggested I try it on. Into the ladies' room I went, slipped the abaya over my head, and proudly walked out. The sister smiled and said it looks great on you but there's only one problem. Dumbfounded, I asked what was wrong. I was so eager to own my first abaya. I had it on backward. Ha! All in all, I dressed conservatively albeit colorfully so a few minor adjustments it was no big deal.

I often wore hats so covering my head (and my now gray hair) was a natural transition. The hijabs (also known as headscarves) came one by one as gifts after I said *shahada* last February. Print hijabs, cotton hijabs, silky smooth hijabs, and several I bought myself. All were so pretty and nice. They piled up week after week until I found myself smothered in hijabs. I felt like a true Muslim woman now. In my boxy one-bedroom apartment, space is tight, especially for a semi-hoarder like me. I can't seem to help myself. I collect "stuff." I hold onto magazines that I'll never read. I just can't resist buying books, especially on sale in thrift shops. I love to read. At breakfast, if the morning paper is late, I'll read the cereal box out of desperation. Do I need another pair of shoes? Probably not but at half price sales and thrift shops it's hard to say no.

Over the years I've learned to live with less primarily because I just don't have the space. I finally re-organized with the help of a wicker basket, moving T-shirts out of the dresser opening space for hijabs. Problem solved? Not exactly. I just cannot seem to keep the scarf drawers neat and tidy despite trying. And trying and trying. What's a girl to do? Yet again, I tidied up my scarf drawers last month, organizing hijabs by color. I was so proud of myself. Classy and stylish, I could open my drawer and pick out a scarf to match my outfit just like that. Wham bam, easy peasy. That lasted maybe a week until the drawers looked like a windstorm blew through them. They're a mess once again. Now that I've become more adept at wearing the hijab I apparently lack at proper storage technique. I could care less about my sock and underwear drawer where I just throw everything in. With hijabs, it's different. They need respect just like our blouses, skirts, and shoes. The right pair of shoes can make or break an outfit.

There's hope for me. A year or two ago, I visited my dear friend Diba who is largely responsible for my conversion. For hijab storage, Diba tightly rolls the scarves much the way I rolled my towel and head for the beach as a youth. The new storage method has already opened-up more space in my drawers. My headwear is sorted out, even if my life isn't quite the same way. Wearing the hijab, however, hasn't always been uneventful. I've been called a raghead and Satan worshipper. Some people glare at me as if I'm a rabid dog. Others have asked me if I'm hot. It's summer time in Phoenix. Everyone is hot, not just me. One day I wore a green print hijab. I thought I looked rather nice. A woman asked me if my hair was green. I chuckled and said that's one I haven't heard before. Yet someone else asked if I had cancer. After the 2016 election, a man driving a pick-up truck noticed me in my hijab as I came out of a grocery store. He sped up in my direction narrowly missing me. It also scared me. Some women stopped wearing the hijab out of fear but I won't succumb to other people's hatred. No woman who covers her head for religious reasons should be fearful.

•

Muslims pray five times a day. I rarely prayed, even though I was raised Catholic. I cut school, skipped mass, and cannot tell you what's in the Bible. My late mother always prayed that I'd return to the church but I never did. Our small apartment sometimes reminded me of a chapel with a large picture of the Last Supper hanging in the living room. Rosary beads and prayer books were scattered throughout. A picture of Jesus stared at me as I ate. Maybe she'd be happy now that I pray five times a day, more than I ever have in my life.

Speaking of prayers, the year 2015 was my first as a Muslim during Ramadan, the holiest Islamic holiday that lasts about a month. Except for Friday nights, when I volunteer at the airport, I attended nightly prayer service at the mosque, also known as Taraweeh, preceded by Iftar. Iftar is a meal to break the sun-up to sun-down fast required for able-bodied adults. Time at the mosque with my Muslim friends became a routine that fulfilled, energized, uplifted, and renewed my soul. After prayers, my faith grew deeper and stronger. I felt closer to Allah, asking again for forgiveness for mistakes of the past. I vowed to spread more harmony, more joy as well as avoid gossip. Chit-chat can hurt others anyway and stain my character so I don't need to do it. I am human though and sometimes make mistakes. I always ask for forgiveness. During Ramadan, sisters welcomed everyone, friends as well as guests. There was no difference among us even though we were a mixed group of Africans, Arabs, Persians, Asians, and Western converts. Islam united us all. Sisters dished up home-cooked meals to elderly or disabled women like me. Although children were sometimes pesky, they really were a delight to be around. School-age girls joined in prayer standing next to their moms. The little ones were an inspiration for the future and it's our collective responsibility to teach them well so they mature into responsible adults as well as fine examples of our faith. Conversation among us was always lively. No one was left out. Afterwards, everyone pitched in to clean up so the room was presentable for prayers.

In the fall of 2016, I ran into car trouble, serious car trouble. The bills stacked up to almost $3,600. Wow, that would've ran up my credit card bill to almost its limit but what could I do? I need a car to get around Phoenix so I had to pay up. Unknown to me, my sisters from the Quran group donated enough money to not only cover the bill but there was money left over. I was flabbergasted. I was in tears when they handed me the envelope with so much cash. No one has ever been that generous to me, not even my family. Several friends donated generously to me over the years and I'll always remember their generosity. But $3,600 was overwhelming. Speechless, I didn't know what to say other than to be humble and thank my sisters. I paid off the car repair bills and donated the extra to Islamic charities. I didn't feel right keeping the extra money.

I am content and satisfied as a Muslim. I found a safe, secure place inside a community of people who care about me. I found my inner hijab. Thank you to all the people who helped and guided me on my journey. You all know who you are. Diba said our encounter that day in the airport was part of Allah's plan. I'm glad it was. I finally arrived after a long, difficult struggle. I didn't do well as a professional writer despite awards, publications in prestigious magazines, and years of trying. The accident ended my chance for a social work career. I tried and failed in the business world. Converting to Islam made me a winner right away. At least I found where I belong. And the accident made me a better person. For that I am so very thankful.

Chapter Twenty-Two
Volunteering in the Muslim Community, Helping Hands for Relief and Development

Now, what would I do on Wednesday since I no longer volunteer at the IRC? Stay home? Not a chance. The over-fifty-five trailer park where I had lived was an active community where many people worked, used the swimming pool, or walked their dogs daily. This place was different, however. Many people seemed content to sit around, watch television or play cards. That was their lifestyle but it wasn't mine; I didn't like staying home more than I had to. I felt bad leaving my little dog Franny home a lot but she slept most of the time. She was content with her two meals a day and a comfortable place to sleep.

I continued my daily workouts at LA Fitness, I had my commitment to homeless animals, and the airport, but, to keep my sanity, I needed to find something to replace the IRC. On days when I had spare time, I stopped by the Helping Hands for Relief and Development (HHRD) warehouse in Chandler to sort and to fold clothes. A global humanitarian agency, HHRD assists needy Muslims in nations like Pakistan, Afghanistan, Jordan, Lebanon, and other nations with used clothing, non-perishable food, shelter, and healthcare. The Chandler office collects gently used clothing and food items like cooking oil, rice, sugar, and lentils. We then package them in boxes for shipment overseas.

One week, I mentioned to the former area manager, Gul S., that I left the IRC. Right away, she said come to the warehouse. That was probably in January 2017 and I've been there ever since. The warehouse is open four days a week, served mostly by volunteers like me. A small group of Muslim women work together every week. During my tenure at HHRD, my experiences have been varied. I might sit in the office one week and no one will come by. Yet on another week, three or more people will come to the warehouse with clothing, food, or cash donations. Donations may be just one bag of clothing or a van full collected from mosques across the city. Some donors will stay to chat for a while. Others drop off the donations and leave quickly. Perhaps they are on the way to work or don't have time. One donor drove all the way from Tucson with a van full of donated supplies. I offer to show the donors around the warehouse and to explain what we do. Some of our donors are from other faiths. They know that we serve Syrian refugee camps and want to help. Their assistance is much appreciated. Now and then, I sit alone in the warehouse and stare at all the donations, in awe our community's strength, generosity, and unity to help our fellow Muslims in Jordan, Pakistan, Bangladesh, or wherever the help is needed. Tears may stream down my cheeks because this is the side of Islam that the media rarely sees. They only present the worst aspects of Islam, not the ordinary every day acts of kindness I see all the time.

HHRD also has a solid connection with the local Church of Latter Day Saints of Jesus Christ, otherwise known as the Mormons. The Mormons are encouraged to perform community service. The local church has a website called Just Serve. Sometimes, HHRD advertises for volunteers on Just Serve and plenty of Mormons, including children, show up at our warehouse to help. We couldn't pack a container without help from the men from the Mormon community. May Allah bless them for their commitment to the Muslim community.

An extremely rewarding aspect about volunteering for HHRD is the camaraderie among my colleagues, many of whom are now my friends. Each week, we laugh and talk as we sort and fold donations. I look forward to my Thursday mornings. We rejoice when 700 boxes of supplies are ready for shipment overseas. That's about how many boxes can be packed into a container. The current manager, Samia H., puts out the word to our many dedicated volunteers and supporters to gather at the warehouse for loading.

Volunteers show up and are ready for an evening of hard work. The container is then driven to the port of Los Angeles. From there, it goes by ship to its next destination. On loading nights, there may be about twenty to thirty people at the warehouse, most of whom are men who are needed to lift boxes. Samia, the manager, takes charge and directs the volunteers so that as many boxes as possible can be stuffed inside. Eager young men and women carry boxes from the warehouse and stack them outside while others hoist them onto the container. It's a backbreaking effort that takes about two hours. Sweaty bodies guzzle down bottled water to stay hydrated because they work up a sweat in the Arizona heat. As Muslims, we break for Maghrib prayer at sunset. I think the guys are also glad to catch a few minutes rest. The women on hand always provide moral support to our industrious brothers for without them we could not accomplish our mission to serve the refugees. Watching men, most of whom I didn't know, load boxes with clothes that I sorted and packed, was rewarding. I often wondered about the refugees who would wear these clothes. What were their lives like? How did they escape from such a perilous situation in Syria? Gaza? Did they make the treacherous journey across the Mediterranean Sea in a flimsy boat? How many relatives and friends did they lose? I listen to news about the war all the time on NPR because I don't have a television. I cry sometimes when I consider how wretched their lives must be after seven long years of war. Women raped, men killed, children left orphaned, and a country in ruins. For what? What has been accomplished? I don't know. I hope that my small effort will make a difference in someone's life.

There are times when I feel hopeless because there is so much war, poverty, despair, and unrest around the world but volunteering at Helping Hands can almost always put a smile on my face. We receive a lot of community support. Volunteers sometimes come in groups from companies or community colleges. Ready, able, and willing men, women, and even children sort and fold clothing into boxes. They may listen to music or talk among themselves. The joy they bring into our warehouse is infectious. Sometimes a lone volunteer drops in to lend a hand. That volunteer could be a college student or someone on their day off. Maybe they'll stay for an hour or two. Perhaps it's a mom on her way to pick up her children from school. The contributions from our community are wide and varied but so much appreciated. My soul is nourished by their caring and kindness.

Samia's schedule is packed. In addition to raising a family, she is a tireless advocate for the refugees, both at home and overseas. She plans fundraising banquets, seeks out hard to find donations, and networks with other agencies to raise awareness about the worldwide refugee crisis. She is always on the move to spread the word about refugees. I admire her dedication and commitment.

I sometimes hear news reports from Syrians saying that the world has forgotten them. No, we did not. Maybe it seems that way because the fighting drags on and on. If I was in Syria living under constant bombardment, starvation, deprivation, and fear, I would likely feel abandoned too. But please know that there are millions of people around the world who care about you. There are thousands of people in Arizona, many of whom I know personally, who worry for your safety. We do our very best to help you out. Sometimes all we can do is pray, but we have not forgotten you. We never will.

·

A friend mentioned that the American Muslim Women's Association served a hot meal twice monthly at homeless shelters. Unavailable on Sundays to assist at one shelter, I had time for the second shelter, a church in Chandler. On the third Monday of every month, AMWA dished out a hot meal to homeless people at a church. Few services were available for single homeless people so a group of churches combined resources and developed a plan. Participating churches in the East Valley cities of Chandler, Mesa and Tempe provide overnight accommodations in their sanctuaries for homeless men and women, and sometimes their dogs. At the church, there are used but clean linens as well as re-usable mattresses. Those homeless people needing overnight accommodation meet at a central location in each participating city. A van driver drops them off at a designated church about 6:15 p.m. and picks them up the following morning about 6:00 a.m. Services are free.

Various community groups like Girl Scouts and AMWA provide hot meals. My friend Nagia does nearly all the cooking. She prepares a rice dish, tossed green salad, and vegetables. From a local grocery, she buys fried chicken and dinner rolls. I arrive early and prepare drinks of iced tea, water, and lemonade that are already available in the church's food pantry. I put out the dinnerware and napkins while we await our guests to arrive. No month is the same. Sometimes, the only volunteers are me and Nagia. In other months, there will be more volunteers, both Muslim and Christian. A member from the church's congregation is always present. Usually, about fifteen to twenty-five homeless people show up. No one is permitted to stay if they show signs of impairment from drugs or alcohol. As the guests enter the church, I notice their haggard looking faces. They carry all their belongings in knapsacks, plastic bags, pillow cases, or suitcases. Their clothes are often tattered and worn. In summertime, they are hot and tired. A few are accompanied by their dogs, often on a flimsy piece of string. Guests stake out a place to deposit their belongings then freshen up in the bathroom, which only has a sink and toilet. There are no shower facilities. When supplies are available, the church puts out a cart filled with toiletries such as soap, shampoo, toothpaste, toothbrushes, and feminine products.

New faces arrive and a few familiar ones show up from the month before. Some guests have jobs, menial positions in hotels, hospitals, or department stores often at minimum wage. They cannot afford the down payment for an apartment which in some cases is one or two month's rent in advance plus a security deposit. Landlords usually charge an extra pet deposit. Now and then, a guest has a disability and comes with a walker or cane. They may have just had surgery or wear a cast due to a broken limb. Some guests are married or a couple. A young woman once appeared terrified of sleeping with strangers. In the four plus years that I've volunteered at the church, I never once heard of any overnight violence. Everyone wants a clean place to rest, a decent meal, and to be off the streets even for a little while.

Social workers are available in each city to help guests secure housing or other essential services. For instance, some homeless people are veterans. They are connected to the Veteran's Administration, a Federal agency, to see what help they can provide. Others are elderly and may qualify for housing assistance because of their age. I met a woman one month who had a dog. She told me that she had obtained a Section 8 voucher, which are used for low-cost housing. There was only one drawback, however. She had to find a participating landlord to accept the voucher within thirty days in addition to one who allowed pets. I never saw the woman again so I assumed her housing search was successful.

Once the food is ready, we ask the guests to line up with women first. We ask someone to lead us in prayer. If no one offers, then a volunteers says a prayer, either Christian or Islamic. Then the food is dished out to hungry folks. As a dog lover, I always carry dog food in my car in case I see a stray or a homeless person on the street with a dog. If a guest has a dog, I offer the food to her. I might sneak a leftover roll to a guest's dog with their permission. The dog is always happy to gobble it up. They suffer too from being out on the street, especially in the long, sweltering summers.

After the meal is served, volunteers sit and chat with our guests. Some are talkative while others wish to be left alone. I respect their wishes. The stories shared are quite similar. They became homeless because of a divorce, job loss, unexpected expenses (usually medical or car related), family crisis, or bad judgment. Only in a few cases did the person admit it was related to drugs or alcohol. I heard from a few guests who lived in dilapidated housing that the buildings were deemed unsafe by local authorities and they had to move without receiving compensation from the landlord. Sudden moves left them unprepared and they ended up homeless. One guest moved to Arizona for a change of venue but came unprepared. The friend who promised him a place to stay reneged. The guest had trouble landing a job and ended up on the streets. The loss of a car caused some guests to lose their jobs. Without enough savings to fall back on, unemployment soon followed. And then came homelessness if there wasn't family help. Public transportation is spotty and unreliable in the Phoenix metro area. Buses run every half hour in many cases. On the weekends, it may be once an hour on some routes. If a person misses a bus connection, he may be late for work. Continued lateness can lead to firing. Losing a car can lead many people to lose their jobs and then their apartments.

Guests appreciate the food we provide and always say thank you. They offer to help clean up by wiping down the tables, sweeping the floor, or collecting the salt and pepper shakers from the tables. Volunteers like me are there to serve them and it is our pleasure to make their lives easier. We see the nagging hardships of life on the street. In the blistering hot summer, homeless people spend their days on the street seeking escapes from the endless heat. At least they can spend the night in a cool, air-conditioned place at whatever church they end up in. I am glad when I hear stories that someone found an apartment or a job. That's a step toward self-sufficiency. There's plenty of paid employees and volunteers in the area to help homeless people get off the streets. The scarcity of affordable housing makes their job so hard but they do their best for our homeless population. For all who serve, I am so thankful as our homeless population never seems to end. I am glad to help even if in a small way.

•

At the end of 2016 or early 2017, Gul, the former area manager for Helping Hands was in a meeting with Wafa, the new owner of the Arizona Muslim Voice as I entered the warehouse. Gul invited me to join them so I did. A post-graduate journalism student at ASU, Wafa was in the office to meet Gul and to learn about Helping Hands for a feature story for the paper. Maybe a week later, I contacted Wafa and told her about my writing experience. She asked me to submit a story.

The first feature I wrote for the *AZ Muslim Voice* concerned an inter-faith Thanksgiving dinner I attended at ASU the month before. Every Thanksgiving, the various faith groups at ASU organize an inter-faith dinner. Everyone in the community is invited. I had attended the year before and thoroughly enjoyed myself among such vibrant guests. What a pleasure to write about an evening of camaraderie, lively conversations, and good food. I covered another story about the Syrian Sweets Exchange at a synagogue. The idea to sell Syrian sweets started in Tucson and quickly spread to Phoenix. Syrian refugee women bake desserts popular back home and sell them to earn extra cash at mosques, churches, synagogues, bookstores, etc. The city of Phoenix also got involved by setting aside free space in a busy down-town skyscraper for a month so that all local immigrants could sell their homemade products. Every time the Syrians held a sale, nearly all the baked goods sold out within an hour. I also attended two meals at a modest cost cooked by Syrian refugees. The fee covered their costs as well as provided them with a tidy profit to help with household expenses. I wrote about vandalism at a Tucson mosque. An intruder broke in and for no good reason ripped up Qurans. The community at large responded to this hateful act by donating new Qurans to the mosque showing the vandal and those who supported him that love always wins. I wrote about Mr. Trump's proposed travel ban, which in essence was a ban on Muslims because the countries he named were primarily Islamic. In fact, I attended one of the protest marches at Sky Harbor airport after the ban was announced. Hundreds of people chanted, carried signs supporting immigrants and paraded up and down outside the main terminal to voice their dismay with the presi-dent's plans. In addition to Phoenix, there were protests at airports, big and small, across the country. I wrote about eco-friendly mosques, big and small. Sadly, not all mosques have caught up to the importance of recycling. Not only would it aid Mother Earth but it would save the mosque money too.

I was delighted to cover a story at my favorite bookstore, Changing Hands. On President's Day in 2017, both stores (Phoenix and

Tempe) donated the proceeds of all sales to the International Rescue Committee. All resettlement agencies including the IRC faced funding challenges resulting from the Trump administration's harsh, punitive immigration policies. Ever since he was elected, he slashed the number of refugees allowed into the USA. I had the pleasure to write about an event during Black History Month linking it with the African American community. There was a lovely celebration in Mesa about world cultures that I wrote about.

Other stories saddened me namely a movie called *Salam, Neighbor* about the bleak lives of Syrians in a Jordanian refugee camp. A group of sisters from my Quran group saw the movie together. Tears streamed down our cheeks as we hugged each other goodbye, realizing how fortunate we were. Syrian women and their families not only escaped from the abject horrors of war but many now lived in squalid, dusty, dirty, and sometimes unsafe camps. I attended a fundraising dinner for the Rohingya, Muslim refugees of Myanmar who fled from the brutality of the Buddhist majority. Like the Syrians, they are packed into overcrowded, unsanitary, and often unsafe refugee camps in Bangladesh. These issues need to be covered so I wrote informative stories as best I could.

During each spring, the MSA at ASU hosts Islamic Awareness Week. There are lectures and movies about various aspects of Islam. In addition, Muslim students set up tables on camps and hand out information about Islam. On same days, visitors to their table will be asked to try on a hijab. Sometimes men will try on the hijab and that's OK. Female students offer henna to anyone who is interested. At the end of the week, students organize a mosque tour for non-Muslims. The grand finale is usually a community service project. I wrote about a weekend course called Portrait of a Prophet that is presented by an out-of-town group called Celebrate Mercy. They host the conference at cities around the USA. Several interesting speakers discussed key aspects of the Prophet's life. For me as a relatively new Muslim, it was an excellent learning experience. I enjoyed meeting and talking with guests and speakers. One of the last articles I wrote concerned the unacceptably high, frightening, and appalling level of violent acts committed since Donald Trump's election in 2016. According to the Pew Research Center as well as the FBI, hate crimes have been on the rise since Mr. Trump's first election. Arson, vandalism, death, and bodily harm against minorities have all been reported.

I enjoyed writing for the *AZ Muslim Voice* but Wafa moved out of state not long after she finished her Ph.D. It was a wonderful chance to keep up my writing skills. I learned a lot as well as met interesting people. I'm sorry it ended.

Chapter Twenty-Three
Final Thoughts

Old age happened so quickly. Seems like the other day when I was a grammar school student bouncing around the play yard at lunch time. To reach the school about three blocks away, I walked either alone or with Jean around the corner. Books weren't banned. Government officials didn't intervene with lessons about slavery. The terms autism or attention deficit disorder weren't yet popular. Children weren't medicated for not sitting still. We were all vaccinated. Parents didn't have hissy fits about it either. Woke? Yeah, I woke up every day. Thankfully, the bomb never dropped. I grew up in the nuclear age and there was always an ever-present fear of the bomb. As a child, I wasn't yet in tune with the growing and often dangerous rivalry between the US and the former USSR. To prepare for Armageddon, we had bomb drills. One by one, with our index fingers pressed to our lips, we filed into large closets where our coats and boots were stored. I always wondered how hiding in the closet would protect us from catastrophe. In my era, there were no mass shootings. Hardly anyone but the police or military owned guns. As city folk, no one went hunting. We didn't kill dinner but bought meat in the store. Childhood obesity wasn't an issue because outdoor activity was so prevalent. We rode bikes, walked the neighborhood to look at rats in the empty lots, and played games in the courtyards that connected our dilapidated buildings.

•

The world has changed so much since January 6, 1994, a major turning point in my life. Blackberry and apple were known as fruits. The term 5G didn't scare some people into torching cell phone towers. A text was a hardcover schoolbook. An app was the beginning of the word application. How did I survive without posting selfies? Not only did I turn out to be a reasonably intelligent person but I earned two college degrees without the benefit of technology. If I wanted the result of 3,456 × 4,738, I did it by hand. In college, calculators were forbidden. We took notes by hand. For real.

What's ahead? Only God knows, not me. I take each day, one step at a time. I am thankful to be in reasonably good health. I can still exercise daily albeit modestly. I live independently and find fulfillment through volunteer work and my community. In the past, during hard times, I sometimes wished that the accident never happened but it did. I did my best to make a new life and hope my readers will be proud. I couldn't have made this incredible journey without the help of my friends and all the people who I've volunteered with. Thank you.

Acknowledgements

Thank you to all the doctors, nurses, and therapists who helped put this Humpty Dumpty back together again after a serious pedestrian car accident on January 6, 1994. If that day had gone on as usual, my life would've chugged along. Maybe it would've been a colossal bore or I might have become a household name for my contributions to society. Who knows?

I appreciate my many friends who stood by me over the years. There's too many to name but I'll mention a few—Maryann, Tui, Julie, Melanie, Mary, Kristin, and the ladies from my weekly Quran group. Thank you to my old writing group—Val, Cindy, Gary, Wanda, and forgive me if I forgot anyone. Although the group didn't contribute suggestions to this book, their comments and suggestions over the years improved my writing. And thank you to the editors and staff at Vine Leaves Press for believing in me and my long recovery.

If the driver swerved that day and missed me, I'd have missed out on so much. I would likely never have become a pet therapist and served with homeless children. My job would've prevented me from spending time as an animal shelter volunteer. The chance to answer the phones for former Gov. Janet Napolitano wouldn't have been possible. Neither would the opportunity to assist refugees. So many volunteer chances that enriched my heart and molded me into a better person would've passed me by. My life is fuller because of the accident. It's doubtful I would've converted to Islam and became part of a vibrant, supportive, and loving community. They're like family. Do I regret the accident? Not at all. I have blessings to be thankful for. So very many.

Vine Leaves Press

Enjoyed this book?
Go to *vineleavespress.com* to find more.
Subscribe to our newsletter: